THE LAST 10LBS

THE LAST 10LBS

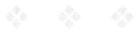

HOW THE LAST 10 HELPED ME TO LOSE 100LBS

Tasha T Turnbull

ISBN-13: 9781981519989
ISBN-10: 198151998X

DEDICATION

This book is dedicated to all the women out there that have tried 478 times in their life to lose weight and just have not found the perfect combination of assistance, tips, gems, and mojo to get from point A to B. Not only do I hope this book encourages you to try again for the 479th time. But on this try, I hope this book empowers you to find the right combination along "The Journey" to push you even further away from point A and get you closer to point B than you ever imagined.

I'd also like to dedicate this book to my friend and client, Nikki Butts. She is one of the strongest women I've met in my lifetime and I love that she is simply not afraid to try again. I'm with you Nikki as we try again, together to assist you with reaching your goals. Game on!

TABLE OF CONTENTS

PREFACE

I HAVE BEEN putting off the idea of writing this book for about five to seven years. Honestly, I always felt I had a story to tell since I started losing weight and maintaining the weight loss for the past 15 years. Nine years of owning a business and conducting fitness training early mornings and late evenings has kept me pretty busy. Therefore, this book had to take a back seat to what I felt was my main attraction. Every day I gave 100% to my business, and by the end of the day, I was way too tired to write a thing. I was in a consistent groove of expanding my business. In addition to helping people reach their goals via personal training, I also run my boot camps, and community fitness events. Focusing on those objectives caused me to overlook the tremendous impact of sharing my journey as motivation to my clients and audiences. Fitness is never just about diet and exercise. It's about everything in between as you are trying to transform your body...It's all about "The Journey."

The weekly conversations I have with my personal training clients, the introductions and closings I have with my boot camp groups, the information I share about my weight loss tips and secrets when speaking to audiences in person or via social media, are times in which I have been able to orally pour into people about realizing the unlocked potential inside of them while on their own journey. We all have the power to transition and transform from our current position. Sometimes, it requires another person's setbacks, and success to inspire you to realize your own capabilities. I wanted to compile all of the information I have shared to help you wherever you are along your fitness journey. I said to myself, "Let me go ahead and write this book, chile."

The Last 10lbs begins with me in elementary, middle, and high school, struggling to accept and love myself, despite feeling that I stuck out like a sore thumb because I was overweight. I developed a large appetite for all foods at a young age. I was and still am greedy. Once I entered college, I took advantage of the easier access to all the junk food life had to offer and ended up gaining an additional 50lbs. Although the food tasted good going down my stomach, my spirit, soul, and health were broken. My self-esteem was low. My weight was high, and I felt my life was not worth living. One day after I left college, I was able to quiet the noise in my head. I realized I still had a chance at changing the trajectory of my life. I decided that I wanted to be an active participant in my life instead of watching everyone else live their lives, while I sat on the side line, chilling. I never knew this new perspective would be the catalyst for me to completely transform my life in just two years.

In Chapter 12, I discuss in detail how I lost the final 10lbs to become a loser of 100lbs total. During the course of this book, I have kept it completely real. I tackle the tough topic of how I fell off track at different points along "The Journey" even after finally realizing my self-worth, losing the first 90lbs and becoming a fitness trainer. *The Last 10lbs* emphasizes the various trying situations I went through which affected my weight gain. I eventually decided to assess, strategize, and implement a plan during each of those time periods, to help me get to a place of peace and weight loss success.

The Last 10lbs is not just a weight loss book for people looking to lose 10 lbs. Think of the term, 'The Last 10lbs' as a metaphor for having difficulty maintaining a healthy lifestyle, wanting to reduce body fat and feel comfortable in your clothes, or desiring to reach your fitness goals after previously starting over 246 times while juggling 24 things daily. Busy work life, family drama, celebrations, raising children, vacations, becoming a BOSS, getting married, grief, divorce, attaining multiple degrees, and opening your own business can all play a significant role in your relationship with food, how active (or inactive) you are, and what focus you have on maintaining a healthy lifestyle. The *Last 10lbs* tells you how I was able to help myself lose 100lbs by finding a unique way to live the healthiest life possible despite a busy schedule and the emotions that come along with a lot of responsibility. I give away a number of tips on what I did to lose the weight and how you can implement them into your own life if you want to lose your own 10lbs. It was a challenge for me to lose weight and maintain the weight loss. Shoot, it's still a struggle, but it can be done. It is up to you to put in the effort of continually loving yourself enough to stop with the excuses and try one more time (or 70 more times) to lead a healthier life. If you're with me, then let me show you what I did and what you can do to lose those last 10lbs, one page at a time.

Special thanks to my friends Ty Cox, Starr Armstrong, and Stephanie Walters for assisting me with the edits for this book. Your support means the world to me. I thank you for your time and effort.

CHAPTER 1

ELEMENTARY & MIDDLE SCHOOL

MY JOURNEY TO losing 100 pounds did not start three, four, or five years ago, it actually started in elementary school. So before I fill you in on how I went from an obese college student to a woman who lost 100 pounds on her own, I gotta take you back to the beginning for a bit. Let me show you where I started to give you a greater perspective on how it is still amazing to me as to how I got to where I am today (both physically and mentally). The grade school years...

It was like clockwork: every day I was teased about my size in elementary school. I mean, every day somebody would say something, and it was mostly the boys in my class. Somehow, I assumed these kids would eventually just give up and focus on something else they thought that was funny – but that never was the case. They just kept coming for me *every* day. I can remember only one other time when there was a girl bigger than me in my class...and that was in the 4th grade. In every other instance, I was easily the biggest girl in my class, so I was

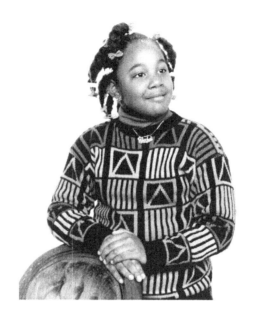

always the target of their jokes. When I discovered that them easing up on me was not gonna happen, I would just hope I would somehow become invisible since I was always so quiet. That didn't work either, and I just kept getting teased on how much bigger I was than any of the other girls. So I just learned to deal with it the best way I knew how: by not saying a dag-on thing. I did not have any swift come-backs for their big-girl jokes and I was not a fighter. Shoot, I did not even hit them with a "that's why yo momma so ugly!" I just looked down at the ground and waited for the verbal assault to end before we finished gym, recess, or lunch. To this day, I cannot figure out why I didn't speak up for myself – not even once! I wasn't one of those loud-mouthed kids: I stayed to myself, got good grades, and kept quiet. Unfortunately, this "silent Susan" approach was something I applied regardless if kids were criticizing me or not. To make matters worse, I did not have a real friend during those years to take up for me and to come back with a joke for them, so I just took it all in, like a big girl (pun intended). I mean, yes, it was true – I was a big girl. But I could've at least spoken up for myself, you know?

I should have told my parents about how I was getting teased in school but I didn't. I did not tell anyone because I was embarrassed about how big I was. Telling my parents meant that I had a problem with my weight and I did not want to talk about that to a soul! Despite me being overweight as a child, preteen, and a teenager, my parents never really brought up the issue to me. For as long as I can remember, my mother has struggled with her weight, and I felt that her issues with weight decreased her ability to assist me with losing weight. She would throw in comments from time to time like "you don't need another plate of food," but that was pretty much the extent of her guidance. My father was in and out of the house when I was young. He was in the Navy, so he would be gone for months at a time, and then he and my mother eventually divorced when I was in 5th grade. My father and I never discussed any of my serious issues growing up; and that also applied to my health issues. The lack of input from my parents about my weight left me further at a loss on how I felt about myself and what I should do to lose weight. I did not speak up for myself when talking to my peers, and I continued to suppress my thoughts when it came to my parents as well. So approaching my mom about the subject was simply not an option. I decided, "I'm just gonna ride this one out by myself and see how it plays out." Truth is, that was not a good option at all because it was killing me inside and I just continued to let it eat away at me. I left elementary school feeling powerless and with incredibly low self-esteem.

When I got to middle school, things were pretty much the same. The jokes got even worse towards me because as we got older, the kids developed a larger vocabulary to use when "joking" about my weight. On the bright side, since we had to change classes in middle school, I did not have to see the same people all day long. Also, there were larger girls and boys than me in middle school, so I was not teased about my weight every day like I was in elementary school. Even though I was not made aware of my weight all the time, I was still sick of my size. To make matters worse, the decrease in fat jokes in middle school were complimented by the jokes made by a girl at the Girls Club. I had attended the Girls Club since I was in elementary school and I loved it! We danced (loved!), played sports (love, loved), cooked, and created arts and crafts. Even though I was as overweight as they come, I was very much an active little girl who loved the outlet the Girls Club provided for me. I loved dancing, playing sports, and performing; I just did not like how I looked while doing it.

Any-who, I absolutely loved going to the Girls Club every day. Going there every day while being an over-weight child, however, came at a price once this new girl started coming, whom I'll call "Tonya." Tonya joked me so badly every single day and I did nothing about it. I just tried to stay out of her way. She was not bigger than me, she was actually quite the opposite. She was a slim girl who had pretty, silky hair and was liked by all the kids at the club. I totally used to envy how slim Tonya was and how all of her clothes fit her so neatly. She had perfect, smooth brown skin and she could eat 6 Otis Spunkmeyer cookies at a time and 2 bags of salt and vinegar potato chips just like the rest of us kids and she never gained weight. Ughhhh, she got on my nerves about how she was so perfect! She was just so pretty… a pretty girl who had decided to make my life absolutely miserable. I remember one week I got called "jigglers" by her way too many times, and I had had enough. She teased me so badly, I told my mom I did not want to go to the Girls Club for a whole week. I had gone to the Girls Club religiously for years, so it was quite a shock to my mom when I told her I did not want to go. When she asked why, I simply said, "I just want a break, that's all." My mom never sus-pected anything, so she did not probe me any further. So I stayed at home and was bored to death for the entire week. When I went back to the Girls Club the following week, Tonya picked right back up with the fat jokes and I absolutely couldn't believe it. She never let up until we got too old to attend the club. I left that summer feeling so sorry for myself: I was pitiful. Since Tonya was my standard of beauty as a child, I was failing miserably as a human. My life pretty much sucked and there was nothing I could do about it. In middle school, I just wanted to be accepted by my peers. I did not need to be the best dressed, the most popular, the fastest person to run, or the best dancer. I just wanted to like myself and for other people to like me as well.

After the end of 8th grade, I met my best friend Ty at the Boys and Girls Club and we were inseparable for the rest of the summer. Truth be told, I met some other friends in middle school like my friend Tyra who was very sweet as well, and my friend Wendy. However, Ty was just the perfect friend that I needed. I was just amazed at how she wanted to be such a good friend to me even though I was overweight. She was also very direct, straight to the point, and told you just how it was, but in a caring way. She was the complete opposite of me and I was cool with it. I was so down on myself that I did not allow myself to believe that overweight people could have real friends, and Ty was a true friend. To be honest, I also envied that Ty was small. She always had the best clothes, the newest Jordan's at the start of every school year, and regardless if she ate a whole pizza from

Chanello's, her legs never resembled tree trunks like mine. I was jealous of her, but I never felt intimidated. She was always down to earth and never brought up my weight because she didn't see it. She saw me as a friend, and I was so thankful for her every day. We are still besties to this day.

Becoming official best friends with Ty made me feel really good, but our friendship did nothing to help me lose weight or to make me feel better about myself, overall. Despite the negative feelings I harbored about myself for several years, I did not know how to lose weight nor did I have any sense of urgency to seek out a successful way to lose the weight. The weight did not stop me from being active, though. I remember my mother signed me up for gymnastics classes towards the end of elementary school, and I participated for about 4 years. My mother signing me up for gymnastics at that time was the equivalent to me winning $3,426.42 right now. I was psyched! I loved going on the balance beam, performing the floor exercise, and just moving and shaking my chunky little body. My family is Panamanian, so I grew up listening to salsa, calypso, and reggae on a weekly basis. With all that music flowing out of the speakers and that Panamanian blood flowing through my veins came a whole lot of dancing. From as early on as I could remember, I used to dance up a storm any chance I could. Whether it be salsa music, reggae, Janet Jackson, J.J. Fad's Supersonic, or MC Hammer, I broke it down hard. Despite all of the activity I was engaged in those years, it was not enough to overshadow the amount of food I was eating and desserts I was sneaking in when my mom wasn't looking. My weight continued to increase.

CHAPTER 2

LOST BUT NO WHERE TO TURN

I WAS SO nervous about going to high school for fear of being teased about my weight. I knew there were more kids in high school than in middle school, so I figured I would get ganged up on by more kids at one time – as you can imagine, I was very nervous for the first day of school. I wanted to blend in as much as possible, and luckily for me, baggy clothes were in style. I begged my mother to buy me a bunch of Nautica shirts, Polo shirts, sweat shirts and the flyest Nike's she could afford to purchase. I loved anything Nautical-related at the time, so a lot of my wardrobe consisted of Nautica. I got my hair done in a bunch of Shirley Temple curls in the front and a French roll in the back. I just *knew* I was fly, chile. I just hoped I would be fly enough to avoid a beat down the first day of school. Ty was a true friend to the end who would fight anybody that tried to start some mess with me, but since we lived in different neighborhoods, had different classes, lunch periods, and study blocks, I knew I would be on my own. The first day of school came and I walked to the bus stop. As I got there, I saw my friend Wendy and was relieved to see a familiar face in the crowd of newbies, but my heart was still beating so fast as I sat in the seat for the 10-minute bus ride to school. Once the bus pulled up to Booker T. Washington High School and I stepped inside the building, I felt like I was kind of in a state of shock. It felt like there were over 1000 kids in the school. I spent a lot of time walking up and down stairs to classes, getting to know my teachers, and just figuring out where I was supposed to go. In the end, I did not get banked and no one joked me, so it was a successful first day for me. I loved high school – there were a whole bunch of older boys and I met new girlfriends. I loved it! I just didn't love myself or how I looked.

My eating patterns increased in high school. The size of my portions got larger and I ate more junk food, like chips and cookies, on a daily basis. What saved me from becoming seriously obese is that my love for being active tended to increase as well. I played sports, which kept my weight mainly in the moderately overweight category. I was 5'7 so being over 200 pounds did not look terrible compared to if I was 5'3. Plus, there were kids bigger than me in high school so that provided me the mix I needed in order to go under the radar of being joked on as much as I was in elementary and middle school. In high school, I stayed very active playing on the basketball team and soccer team. Since we practiced 5 times a week, I just knew once I got on the team I would lose weight. I was so excited I was finally going to know what it felt like to be a normal person.

Despite all of that activity on a weekly basis, I barely lost any weight. I was heartbroken once I finished that first year of high school – all of that dag-on huffin' and puffin' for nothing! I mean, I would be in the heat all day after school doing soccer drills or getting home late in the winter practicing how to be a better rebounder, all the while thinking about how it was going to help me lose weight. Through all the practices, basketball games, and soccer games, I might've lost 5 pounds. Every single morning, I would stand up and look down at my legs to see if they got any smaller. I always checked my legs because they were the biggest thing on my body. And every time I looked down, they were still bigger than two turkey legs people eat at the carnival. I was a hot mess. I learned in high school that my body did not respond favorably solely to physical activity. I had to combine healthy eating and physical activity in order for me to see some results, but this strategy could not work for several reasons. First, I just was not informed and disciplined enough at that age to carry out that plan. Second, I could work out all day but was extremely lazy when it came to putting in effort to change my eating habits. Shoot, food tasted too good to change! Lastly, throughout all the criticism I received in grade school and my internalization of these jokes, I became broken. I was so down on myself that I could not imagine having the mental strength to change how I felt about myself and, therefore, my body. So despite the strenuous workouts, I continued to get bigger in high school and became even more uncomfortable in my own skin.

My bootleg attempts to lose weight in the summer of middle school and high school were all over the place. It was the 90's and I loved to be active, so I had all of the Jane Fonda, Tae-Bo, Denise Austin, Step Aerobics, and Buns of Steel videos you could imagine. I inconsistently used the tapes anywhere between two to four days a week. I religiously performed all of the fitness workouts that came on TV on ESPN in the mornings. I also had access to weights, jump ropes, a stationary bicycle, and a step bench at home, and I used all of them on a weekly basis as well. I had no problem with moving or getting sweaty, so I hit it hard when it came to the workouts; however, the food was where I had the difficulty in getting my life together. In the 90's, Slim Fast and Nutrisystem were heavily advertised as supplements to drink for weight loss. I asked my mom to buy them for me. I drank the shakes off and on for several months, and I could not stand them. I ate PowerBars and they tasted worse than the shakes. I also snuck and bought weight loss pills from GNC. I remember going into the store and buying some fat burners and being unsure if the guy would sell them to me because I was only 13 years old. I had heard plenty of times that fat burners were not safe to use, but I was desperate so I bought them. I drastically wanted results but was also scared that I'd die from taking them, so I stopped after taking them for 3 days. Incidentally enough, I purchased weight loss pills about 3 times within a 12-month period but never even got through half the bottle; I was too afraid of what could happen to me. I tried the cabbage soup diet but that made me stay in the bathroom for most of the day, and I did not have time for all of that. I started to eat those fat free potato chips that were made with Olestra, but again, started to spend a lot of time chilling on the toilet stool, so I gave up on that one as well. With all of the weight loss fads I tried, I never stuck with them for longer than a few weeks. My weight loss efforts were failed attempts at fixing a problem that had nothing to do with pills and shakes. I was not motivated to perform real transformation in my body. During this time in my life, nothing could overshadow the power of food and how much of it I was consuming on a daily basis.

EXTREME WEIGHT LOSS TACTIC: STARVATION

Getting good grades, making friends, chasing boys, and even playing sports came second to food. My main focus in life was eating, Ok! Rice was a staple in our household and it stuck on me like glue. My mother always served a vegetable on our plate but it was always a small portion, compared to the star of the show, rice. Being the product of 2 Panamanian parents, rice was eaten for dinner about 6-7 days a week, and the portions were large. The other day of the week we had spaghetti. You couple this with the fact that I would eat potato chips and/or dessert following my meal, that's how I became a women's size 14 in high school. Our house contained junk food just like everyone else's, but I had no control when it came to the size of my meals or snacks. Two servings of potato chips would not be enough for me. Nah, I would need to eat the whole bag to be satisfied. I could not eat just one Little Debbie Cake, oh no!! I would polish off the whole 8 pack of brownies within 10 minutes flat. After I finished my sophomore year in high school, I was so sick of myself being this fat blob that I had had enough. It was the summertime and I did not have much going on – I was just sitting at home watching TV. After trying Slim Fast shakes for breakfast followed by Tae-bo workouts with Billy Blanks in the morning – a routine that was not cutting it – I simply decided to starve myself... for the entire summer. I ate once a day and on some days, I ate nothing. I'm not sure how much weight I lost, but looking back, I would have to say I lost anywhere between 30-40lbs. Once I lost the weight, I just knew I would instantly feel happy because I was so small. I just knew all the boys would like me and I would be able to wear cute dresses and not get joked by kids. But honestly, I felt no change. I was not happier and I did not feel better about myself. Instead, I was extremely tired and I had no energy. After I lost the weight, I continued doing the same thing I was doing while I was bigger, sitting on the couch watching TV. I lost so much weight that I even lost my period for 2 months. I had no idea at the time how much stress the extreme weight loss put on my body. Instead of feeling happy, I was lethargic, confused, and still unsure about the best way to lose weight.

Once it was time for my junior year of high school, I was ready to show off my new body. I pretty much wore the same baggy clothes as before but I was eager to see if people would notice. Everyone noticed that I lost weight and wondered what I did to lose it. I simply responded, "I cut back on eating so much," never saying I completely stopped eating and was tired as I don't know what. My soccer coach even joked around when she saw me and asked, "Did you start smoking crack?" My weight loss was a shock to everyone and I thought it was so cool. But honestly, I was hungrier than 2 nuns on the run and I did not feel good about myself. I did not feel prettier: I felt empty and baffled about how I was supposed to keep this weight loss charade up and not die from starvation. So when I got home from that first day of school, I was home alone and I made a Duncan Hines vanilla cake with vanilla frosting. After I made the cake, I just stared at it for a few minutes. I had not been this close to cake in 3 months. I ate 2 pieces and then I just sat in front of it for another hour. After that, it was a goner: I ate 3/4ths of the entire cake. This was the starting point of me going back to overeating for the rest of my high school years, gaining all 40 pounds back.

My relationship with food has been horrible for as long as I can remember. I abused food and looked to it as a form of enjoyment, primarily because it tasted good and I did not like what else was going on in my life. I looked to food for love, support, guidance, friendship, stability, and trust. Although I made friends, had parents who loved me, got good grades, and was involved in a ton of extra-curricular activities in high school, I was very hard on myself because I felt like I did not fit in. I could not fit into the clothes in the junior section at the mall and that was depressing. These clothes were made for everyone my age, so since I was unable to fit them, I felt that something was wrong with me. I was really mad that my legs were so big and could not fit into those cute plaid short skirts all the girls were wearing. When I played basketball, I always wore a t-shirt underneath my jersey. When people asked me why I wore an extra shirt, I said it was because I don't like the sweat to hit my skin while I was playing ball. But in actuality, I wore the t-shirt so people could not see the size of my arms. To make matters worse, I also wore a size 10 shoe so my feet stuck out and it was hard for me to find shoes in my size. As for my face, I felt like I was a 'Plain Jane.' I did not feel like I was ugly, but I never felt pretty either. I mean I was just plain mad at myself from head to toe. And you know I validated these thoughts because I never received any compliments from people. You know how some people are known for always dressing so stylishly or for having pretty hair, or for having pretty skin or being the best player on the team, or maybe even having a coke bottle shape? Yeah, none of those compliments floated my way and I wanted that type of attention.

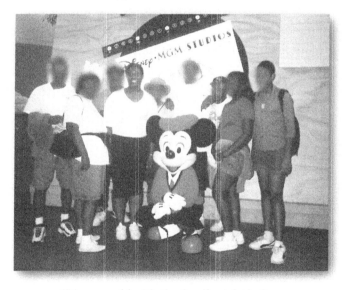

(Disneyworld with the family right before
college started in the fall.)

How I appeared to everyone else was such a big deal in my high school years. I mean that's what girls do – we obsess over clothes, hair, and boys, right? Well, for some reason, my obsession turned into self-hate. When the teasing from other people fell off, I picked it right up and ridiculed myself every day because I was bigger than most of the girls and I did not like the way I looked. I did not need anyone else to tease me ever again in life because I became my own worst critic. I had no idea what to do about the negative feelings I developed for myself, so they just stayed bottled up inside of me.

Since I'd been living and looking this way for the past seventeen years, I accepted it as truth. And that is just the life went for me for the rest of high school.

CHAPTER 3

THE COLLEGE YEARS WERE AN AWAKENING

It was time for college and I was nervous and excited at the same time about how my life would change. Since I was a first-generation student entering college, I was not able to get advice about the college experience from my mother, father, grandparents, aunts or uncles. I just mostly talked to my friends about it. I knew I wanted to major in business in college, so it was important that the school I attended had a stellar business program. I was not sure what type of business I wanted to obtain, I just knew I wanted to run my own business one day.

I ended up applying to 3 schools based on their business schools: The University of Virginia (UVA), Hampton University, and Howard University. All 3 schools accepted me, so I was psyched. Go Tash! However, once I received my acceptance letters, I quickly learned that Howard and Hampton cost 2 arms, 6 legs, and a chicken biscuit for me to attend. Since my parents could not afford to pay for my college, I was left with the hefty burden of paying for college on my own if I wanted to attend. I didn't have some rich uncle or grandmother who lived in New Mexico or savings bonds saved up in my name to cash out to pay for college. If I wanted to attend Howard or Hampton, it all depended on me, and for a 17-year-old teenager, that was a huge responsibility for me to take on. Shoot, I would still be paying those 4 years back this very minute as it would end up costing me over 100k to attend both of those schools. Even at a young age, I looked at debt as financial enslavement, so it was a no-brainer that I would attend UVA. My parents and I did not even have a real discussion about it – there was nothing to discuss. UVA provided grants and scholarships and they even recommended additional scholarships for me to apply for that didn't even come from the school. The only thing my mom paid to the university was the cost of my books in my first and second year. So yeah, without question, I was going to be a UVA Wahoo. I was psyched when I got accepted into the University of Virginia. I mean, me?!?! I did my research and based off of several national polls, UVA was always ranked as one of the top 3 public universities in the entire country (and still is to this day), so I was honored to be accepted. I was the first one in my immediate family (and a large part of my extended family, on both sides) to attend college so it was a big deal for me to attend this school. Their business school (The McIntire School of Commerce) was stellar, to say the least, so I was ready to push forward and receive a degree in Management Information Systems.

Since I was the first one in my family to attend college, UVA thought it would be a good idea for me to attend a week long student education program the summer before school started. When I arrived, most of the kids in this program were African American and our families were on the lower income side of the spectrum, so I guess this was their way of preparing us for what was to come. When I arrived on campus, I realized it was a totally different culture. Coming from predominantly African American elementary, middle, and high schools to a predominantly white school, the transition was a hard one for me. That's especially true given everything else that comes along with going to college, like the coursework being so difficult, being around people from so many different cultures, and my already-low self-esteem. It was a difficult transition for your girl to handle. I saw first-hand how some white people were just plain racist, and it was quite shocking. But more than anything, I was still at a complete loss on how to deal with my weight ballooning into the 200 lb. territory.

You ever say to yourself, "Ok, this summer or this month I'm gonna buckle down and lose this weight once and for all!" Well, I said that the summer after I graduated from high school. I've got 2 months to get under 200 lbs and college is the perfect starting point for my new body and new start into being an adult. Well, the problem with that scenario is I had no game plan, no real motivation, and no desire to take charge of losing actual weight. So beforc you know it, days passed and it was time for me to officially start school.

It was move in day for the start of my college life at UVA. August had come pretty quickly and with no weight loss in sight, my strategy was to not draw attention to the fact that I was overweight. So the natural idea for me was to wear sweat pants on move-in day (Go figure!). Wearing sweatpants was my plan and I was sticking to it no matter what! Now, Charlottesville, VA around this time in August was easily 90 degrees. People had on tank tops, shorts and flip flops since it was so hot, and you spent most of the day going up and down stairs moving in your furniture. Well, that thought process didn't carry over to Tasha! I was so self-conscious about my weight that I decided to stick to my original plan and wear a long-sleeve gray t-shirt and my favorite dark blue sweat pants to lug suitcases and furniture up and down stairs in the heat. Not only did this draw attention to me, but I was burning up! Definitely not one of my smartest moves.

I did not have a car in high school so my food intake was more or less controlled by what my mother brought in the house or what I got in school. Heading away to college and being far away from home meant I had more access to food. Looking back, my most dramatic increase in weight came in college because I had any and all types of junk food available to me at any time of the day. Instead of gaining the freshman 10, I gained the freshman 50.

We had access to cafeteria food at the usual meal times, and boy did they bring out the good stuff. Monday through Sunday I could eat Belgian waffles for breakfast, pizza for lunch, and lasagna for dinner. There were so many choices available at each meal that I could not believe it. When you are at home, you eat what is prepared by your parents. So it was a drastic change for me to have so many options and add-ons. I could get a huge piece of cornbread or the biggest brownie or cookie to my heart's content at every meal. Now don't get me wrong, there were healthy options available to eat as well. Ninety-five percent of the time, however, I went with the greasiest, sweetest, or saltiest food in sight. In addition to the regular meals of breakfast, lunch, and dinner served at the cafeteria, the university had what is called "after hours." After-hours food at the cafeteria was code for any and all the late night junk food you could imagine. In addition to getting fast food items at the cafeteria, it didn't help that you didn't even have to leave campus to eat at Chick-Fil-A. The Tree House was also a place on grounds that sold junk food like Pizza Hut pizza and cheesesteaks, and it was open until 11pm every night. Last but not least, there was even a convenience store on campus where you could get items like candy and Ben and Jerry's Ice Cream until 12am. The worst part about all of this is that you did not need to have cash to purchase any of these items: you just swiped your student-ID card and it was taken out of your semester account. Since there was no limit on what you could purchase, I ate to the max every day. I couldn't believe I could eat all of the best things in the world whenever my stomach made room for it (aka, got larger to keep taking in all of the excess food). From the moment I stepped on grounds, I was in food heaven.

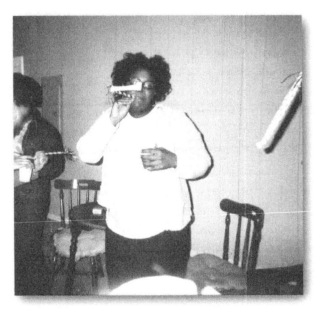

Most of my friends ate the same food as I did and we all gained weight in college; however, I always felt the effects more from a health standpoint because I was obese prior to arriving. As I worked to embrace college life, my physical activity level dropped. Playing organized sports in high school kept my weight at a somewhat maintainable level, but I stopped playing sports when I got to college. I decided against joining an intramural sports team for several reasons.

- One, the level of play of UVA's intramural teams was higher than what I was used to playing at Booker T. and I would not be able to keep up with those girls.
- Two, the intramural sports teams competed just like the national teams and I would miss too many days of school to be able to keep up with my classes.
- Three, the coursework at UVA was rigorous.

I struggled in most of my classes to get good grades because the difficulty and amount of coursework at UVA was much higher than what I was accustomed to in high school. There was no way I was going to let this wonderful opportunity pass me by without getting a degree at UVA. So I buckled down and worked really hard to get good grades in school… I just made sure I didn't pass up any of the junk food while I was at it.

During my 3rd and 4th years of college, my friend Sahrah and I actually started to hit the gym on grounds once or twice a week. The amount of energy I expended during those workouts, though, were nothing in comparison to how many calories I was taking in daily, seven days a week. Although getting to the gym twice a week took effort, it was a poor attempt I made to try to lose weight. I still did not do anything to change the wild eating habits I developed in college. The jeans I started my 2nd year off with

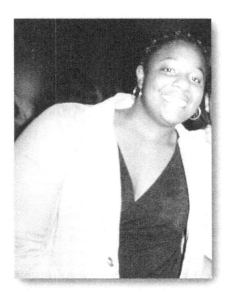

no longer fit by the time I graduated. It wasn't that I just could not zip them up, I could not even get the jeans up my thigh. Boy was that an eye opener! Even though no one could tell I gained so much weight because I wore a lot of big clothes, it hurt me to my core.

Although I dealt with self-hate issues all throughout high school, I never felt that me being overweight was thrown in my face or made me feel like the odd man out. I still was able to develop friendships, had a boyfriend, loved to dance, was the co-editor of our high school's newspaper, played basketball and soccer, was in the honors society and volunteered in several organizations. In college, it was more difficult to cultivate those types of relationships and successes because my self-doubt grew each year that I gained weight, coupled with the fact that I didn't look like the majority of students, so I didn't feel completely comfortable opening up to people. I was never an uber social person to begin with and that personality trait grew stronger in college.

On the other hand, you would not think since I went to a predominantly white school, that I would learn about myself. The truth is, it was the complete opposite. I double-majored in Economics and African and African American studies so I was learning a ton about black culture, black history and black people within the Diaspora. The curriculum for a major in African and African American was extensive, with classes focused on historic (and unspoken of) Black women in United States, Africans in Brazil, Africans in the Caribbean, Democratic Republic of Congo, South Africa (huge), Slavery, During Reconstruction, and specific African kings and queens that I was not privy to in grade school. The pride I experienced by learning so deeply about people who looked like me also created a strong desire inside me to stop relaxing my hair. Although being natural is quite the norm these days, it was a very foreign concept (and considered quite weird) in 1999 and 2000. I would not say this was an ideal time to make such a drastic decision considering I was already feeling very fragile about my body image, but, nevertheless, I went for it.

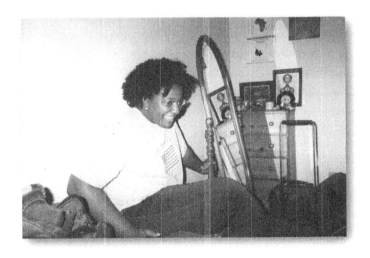

Even though I attended a predominantly white insti-
tution, there were over 30,000 people who attended
The University. With a 12% population of black people
on campus, that meant that there were over 3000 black
people on university grounds, which ·was way more
people than I ever attended school with before, even
in all 12 years of secondary school. With all the black
people on campus, however, I still stood out from the
majority as well as the majority within the black community on the grounds because of my size and complexion. Generally speaking, you had to be slim, of a lighter
complexion and have long hair to be deemed as attractive by the guys in school. Considering I was 0 for 3 in
all of these categories, my dating life sucked. Blending
in as opposed to standing out is what got you favorable

attention in college. And since I did not fit the status quo, I was never asked out on a date by a guy at UVA, which was a far cry from my dating life in high school. I didn't need to have 5 guys lined up to date me, but a date here or there, flirting, and male attention are pretty typical occurrences for girls in college. I experienced none of that and it was depressing. Now don't get me wrong, I came in to college with friends and my BFF Ty from high school, developed new friendships, had a ton of fun breaking it down at the dances on campus, and the basketball and football games were crazy fun. But I did not open up a ton to trying new things – I just was not self-confident enough to want more for myself. I started to turn inward and just focus on getting through these four years done the quickest way possible. College was a self-esteem killer. By the end of those four years, I was the heaviest I've ever been in life and was also the most depressed I've ever been. I was the first person to graduate from college in my immediate and my extended family that I grew up knowing first-hand. It should have been an awesome time for me, but the truth was that it wasn't that big of a deal. My achievement was overshadowed by the fact that I was the heaviest I had ever weighed in my life. To make matters worse, all of the hard work I put in for the past four years to graduate from that school and I could not even get a freaking job. I mean, *really?*

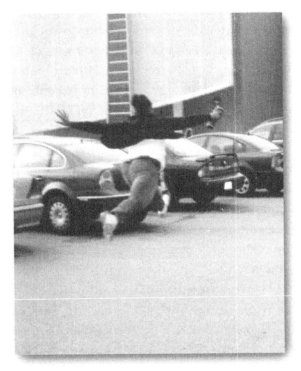

(No matter my size, I've never let it stop
me from being an active person.)

CHAPTER 4

GET YOUR LIFE TOGETHER, TASHA

I FINISHED COLLEGE with a double major degree in Economics and African and African American Studies. It was a great accomplishment that got me no freakin job. I was so pissed off! I was always told to go to college and you will be rewarded with a great job and money. Needless to say, I knew once I finished college I would be able to purchase a Lexus and a townhouse once I graduated (I did not want a detached house because I did not want to the cut the grass: ain't nobody got time for that!). No one told me what really was going to happen was I was going to work my butt off for four years only to return to live at my mother's house and stare at the wall. Furthermore, during this time period, none of my clothes fit and I only could wear my sweat pants, big sweaters and big t-shirts. I continued to eat because, well, I did not have anything else popping off in my life. In essence, my life felt pretty crummy. A few signals started to rise during this time which caused me to evaluate whether I needed to take action and regain control of my life.

After a few months at home, physical and mental changes started to develop that would have a long-standing impact on my life. On a random Tuesday evening, I was at home chillin' and watching one of my favorite shows, *Girlfriends*, when all of a sudden I started crying. I felt completely fine prior to this outburst and nothing dramatic occurred in the episode, but I just started crying. There was no tragedy that had recently struck me, my friends, or my family, so I was confused and unsure how to proceed. Nevertheless, I just wiped my tears and continued on with my life. About a week later, I was pumping gas into my car at the gas station and ended up in tears. Another night, I was at the club with my girls, Ty and Starr, and then all of a sudden I started crying. We had to immediately leave the club. To combat these random bursts of tears, I tried to take deep breaths, pray more, and even had the elders pray over me at church and I still felt like crap. And I mean these just weren't tears, there was crying, loud sobs, and snot that could last over 10 minutes. I had no idea what was wrong with me and it was so weird because I've never been a big crier. Yet, there were these epic ugly cries coming out that felt like they've been trapped in me for some time. I finally told my mom about it after one day I went to use the bathroom and I just started crying on the toilet for no reason. I thought she was going to look at me like I was crazy (because that is how I started to feel about myself), but being the awesome mom she is, she offered me words of encouragement, assured me I would be fine, and said we need to see a therapist. A week later, my mother and I head in to see a therapist. I attend the meeting alone while my mother sat in the waiting room. After asking me several questions, the therapist told me I had Major Depressive Disorder and I was like, "Well what in the hell's bells?!"

So I started going to therapy on a weekly basis. I feel like once I found out I was depressed, it made me even *more* depressed. You ever been crying about something and then someone comes up to you and asks you "What's wrong?" and that causes you to start crying even harder? Yep, that was totally me trying to understand this whole depression situation; it caused me to feel lower than 50 feet below the ground. The best way I can describe how depression impacted me is how it was described in that Cymbalta commercial back in the day. You remember the commercial for the depression medication that showed a girl sitting on a bench and then a cloud comes over her, it starts to rain on her head and she starts to look sad? Well, yeah, that was totally me. It was as if this dark cloud would come over me and I felt horrible, and nothing could get me out of it until the cloud decided to pass on its own and ruin someone else's life for the next few days. These major depressive episodes would come and go for the next 6 years. I don't think therapy resolved my depression as I still experience depressive moments from time to time. The chemical imbalance that occurred in my brain, which resulted in depression, still remains, but it's just not at the level that it was once I left college. What I think helped me during these dark days was speaking with someone on a regular basis who was unbiased and was there to help me process my feelings. I was able to open up and talk about my weight, my relationship with my mother and father, my experiences at college, and feeling like a failure because I was the smartest unemployed person that I knew. I bottled these situations up inside me for the past 23 years and discussing them with someone is what was needed to help me out more than anything. I actively participated in seeing a therapist for about 2 years. I also took a low dose of medication for depression about 11-12 months within that 2 year time period.

Another trigger that signaled a need for change was my blood pressure. I'd been overweight my entire life, and ever since I was a child, my blood pressure would always register as borderline. The nurse would need to take my pressure at least 3 times to get it to read somewhat normal. Heading to the doctor's office always made me so nervous; not for fear of being diagnosed with strep throat or the flu and needing to be on medication, but because he might say something about my weight. So once we got to the doctor's office, I always avoided the doctor's face hoping she would not say I would need to be on medication because I was too big for my age and I needed to lose weight. She would just call out my weight and blood pressure and state that they were on the higher side. She never said that I needed to reduce my blood pressure and lose weight, but deep down I knew that was her concern and I needed to do something about it. I just did not know how to change it. I knew most of the people in my family had high blood pressure and were on medications for it. I did not want to be on medication, but I'd been dealing with this health concern for so long it became my uncomfortable normal and I was not strong enough to change "normal" after all of those years. In my 20s, I also started to develop low back pain and did not have the slightest idea why this started. I was only 22 years old, so I had difficulty figuring out why my back started hurting and I did not lift anything heavy except for plates of chicken wings and rice. Upon doing research online, I learned that the heavy thing I was lifting was my own body weight; it was putting pressure on my lower back. I never saw the doctor about it for fear he would tell me I needed to lose weight.

During this time period, my weight got up to around 235lbs and I was sick of myself. There were too many moving parts taking place in my life that I felt like I had no control over. I felt like I needed to do something to change how I felt about my weight, my health, and how I felt about myself in general. But I was at a complete loss for changing who I was. I noticed myself in the mirror – I knew what I looked like and that my clothes were not fitting. I felt that I was too young to experience depression, high blood pressure, and low back pain. I knew all of these issues stemmed from me being obese, yet I had difficulty accepting that all of these things were happening to me. I was always a by-the-book type of person. I learned early on that working hard, getting good grades, and going to college would provide you with happiness and a great job. Well, I followed that plan to the T and I did not end up with any one of those. I mean, was I lied to all of these years about the importance of getting a 4-year degree and how that equaled success? Because I sure did not feel successful. I was overweight (now weighing over 250lbs) and pissed off about my post-college situation, single with no guy in sight,

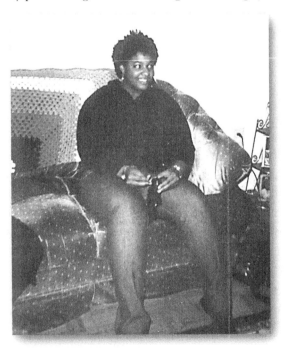

I could not fit into most of my clothes, I was labeled as clinically depressed, I was fed up with how I looked, I was unemployed, and I lived with my mother. In Tasha terms, I might as well have been a death row inmate.

To me, my feelings were 100% validated and I succumbed to them. While I waited for a job to come through, I volunteered at the Urban League in Norfolk for 15 hours a week helping to get other people in the community prepared for job interviews and encouraging young moms to establish a healthy relationship with their kids. I love my people, so I wanted to do something positive for my community with all the free time I had. But the good deeds I committed did nothing to fix the hole that started to fester in my heart. I stayed there for about 12 months, going through the motions of being an overweight, college graduate with no money. I was so disappointed in myself that no one could help pull me out of this fog. So I just ate, volunteered, and felt sorry for myself day after day.

Then one day, I started to analyze myself. No complaining, criticizing, pouting or ridiculing. I started to simply assess what was currently going on in my life. I'd been an emotional wreck for so long, it became hard to step outside my feelings and get a firm grip on how things have played out for me for the past six or seven years. The negatives encapsulated the positives so much that I could not even take one step forward. I'd now come to point where I was tired of feeling stuck. Now do not get me wrong, I was not a toothless, bedridden woman with bad breath and orange tentacles coming out of my hands and feet. But being teased in grade school, finishing college 50lbs heavier than when I started, having no job in sight, and feeling so depressed that I forced myself to put on a fake smile for the people around me was what stuck out. I did not wake up one day and have this big "AHA moment" or this major epiphany that caused me to want to change the way I was living my life. Nah, I would say it was more of a continual accumulation of truths that started to smack me dead in the face, and I began to open my eyes to what was happening to me. My back was against the wall and I felt like I was suffocating. I literally felt that I was choking and breathing at the same time. Have you ever had that feeling? I am responsible for my one-self and I had no control over what was going on. Days were passing me by and I could not find joy in any one thing that was going on. *I was over myself.* I mentally decided on this day that I wanted to lose weight; however, it seemed like I had a fat chance in hell (pun intended) of being a small person. Shoot, I've never been small in my life, ever! All of my pictures (except for when I was an infant) in childhood, high school, college, and post college, were of someone overweight... and, according to BMI standards, obese; therefore, I knew it was highly unlikely that I could really change my physical appearance.

THE NEED FOR FOUNDATION

As you remember, I tried a ton of workout videos, several of those nasty weight loss shakes, worked out at the gym, played sports all throughout high school, and took weight loss pills and never saw a half a pound lost from my body. I even successfully starved myself that one fateful summer, so it was not like I was unaccustomed to putting effort into losing weight. I just lacked 3 skills needed to establish the proper foundation to take charge over my health:

1) The knowledge of how to lose weight in a healthy and permanent manner.
2) The discipline needed to transform my body.
3) The self-confidence and self-love needed to change my weight and body in any significant and permanent way.

These 3 points are key for anyone attempting to lose weight permanently. Additionally, I did not have someone in whom I could confide – someone who had lost weight in the past and/or who could help me develop a plan to lose weight. My weight was always a sensitive and emotional issue to me. When anyone spoke to me about my weight or brought up the topic of weight around me, I would start to get anxiety. I became so nervous when people (whether it be associates, friends or family members) talked about weight that I would automatically put my head down and pray that the focus would not turn to me. It would feel as if my blood pressure would start to boil from within. So I would not dare bring more attention to myself by asking the people who knew me for help with weight loss or telling them that I was going to actively start to lose weight. I mean, what if I didn't lose weight? Then people would think I was a failure, right? I could not bear the possible judgement and questions that would come my way once I said, out loud, that I was going to lose weight.

So I did not say a word to anyone. I knew I would be on this journey by myself and I was okay with that. My anxiety about starting another weight loss "diet" was different this time because I was ready to fully commit to the process, not just the weight loss. My sanity and comfort came from me embracing what I was going to start and The Journey I was about to embark on.

YOU GOT A PLAN, TASHA?

I came to grips with the fact that I was going to be on this arduous journey, and it didn't cause me to panic at all. This was one of the signals that I knew I was sick and tired of being overweight. *I was over myself.* I was completely done with feeling sorry for myself, not liking to look in the mirror, wearing the same 1 pair of jeans and 3 leggings because I didn't want to go to the store and try on clothes that would not fit. I was tired of worshipping and praying to food. I was tired of being engrossed with it. I was sick of envying other people's bodies and not my own. I did not want to just get up and exist – I wanted to *live*. I was tired of living in a fog every day; shoot, I had on blinders for 23 years and could not see a thing. You ever moved through life with blinders on? It's not easy, in fact, it is a pretty hard life to live and I was over it. I knew there was something different flowing within me this time. So what was it, Tasha? I could not put my finger on it. Maybe it was more mojo, juice, fervor, a sense of urgency, and/or an unwavering desire to change what had been holding me back for so long. But the energy I used to have to live a directionless life was transitioning into energy being used for a more purposeful life.

I started to evaluate the 3 skills I would need if I was going to have to lose this weight which were knowledge, discipline, and self-love. I started with what I felt was the easiest of the three to develop: gaining knowledge into a safe and effective way to lose weight. I started doing my own research on the topic of weight loss. The internet was not a big thing at the time, so since we did not have Wi-Fi at my mother's house, I went to the library instead. I read several books on weight loss and found out the two main components you need to change on your weight loss journey: your physical activity and diet. I already knew I needed to get a hold on my food intake and to work out on a consistent basis, but I felt that I needed a better understanding about what impact food plays on how the body is developed in order for me to stick with it this time around. I wanted to lose weight and be healthy. I did not want to lose 40lbs in

3 months (like I did in high school) just to gain 40 + 8 more of those pounds back by the end of the year. I wanted this weight loss to be definite and to stick!

To give a small history lesson on nutrition, the foods we eat are broken down (once they enter the body) into three main components known as macronutrients: carbohydrates, protein, and fat. Carbohydrates provide our bodies with the most energy out of the three macronutrients. Carbohydrates are needed to "ensure that the brain and nervous system function properly as well as helps the body use fat more efficiently. Eating carbohydrates is also the best way for us to obtain dietary fiber," so we want to include them in our diet.[1] There are three important things I didn't realize about carbohydrates before doing my research. First, any type of food that contains carbohydrates means that its chemical make-up is composed of sugar compounds and water, hence the name "carbo hydrate." Two, it does not matter if the food I eat is a fruit, vegetable, starch, or a Twinkie – carbohydrates are pretty much in everything. I thought I was only eating carbohydrates when I was reaching for something sweet, but then I learned carbs were off and popping in savory foods as well. So even when I'm eating my Lays Sour Cream and Onion potato chips post-dinner, 2 cups of rice and peas on Sundays, and pizza on Fridays,

---

1 Copyright © 2003 American Council On Exercise. All Rights Reserved. Reprinted by Permission.

I was still taking in sugar. I was crushed. Complex carbohydrates are a little healthier for you as they contain fiber, can help lower cholesterol, and will release slower into the blood stream so the pancreas does not have to work as hard. So I decided to up my intake of brown rice, sweet potatoes, and whole grain bread. Even though fruit is a simple carb, I decided to keep that in the mix as well because fruit contains so many vitamins, minerals, and fiber that it is too healthy to pass up.

Protein is necessary to "build and repair body tissues, including muscles, ligaments, and tendons. Protein is also important for the synthesis of hormones, enzymes, and antibodies, as well as for fluid transport and energy." Proteins are made up of amino acids that are essential (cannot be made in the body and must be received from food) and non-essential (they are made in the body). Since protein is not stored, we need protein on a daily basis to help the body repair itself from the cell degeneration that happens every day we are alive. From a fitness standpoint, protein is necessary to help repair the body from the muscle fibers that were torn in your previous resistance-training based workout. To help the body repair and for those muscles to grow from your workout, protein synthesis must occur. [2]Protein synthesis cannot occur without some type of stress load being put on the

2 Copyright © 2003 American Council On Exercise. All Rights Reserved. Reprinted by Permission.

body (resistance training), testosterone, and sufficient protein. Lean protein needs to be taken in and I knew I was not getting an adequate amount of protein since I lived off of carbohydrates.

Let me backtrack for a second. By the end of my 4th year in college, I started to do a ton of research on food and what is considered healthy and unhealthy. My research brought me to studies and documentaries revealing the ill-effects of eating animal protein on a regular basis. I learned how companies breed animals in harsh conditions and kill them, but not before injecting them with so many hormones and chemicals. After this unhealthy transformation occurs, the "chicken" heads to the deep fryer before being placed between 2 pieces of bread for lunch or on my plate for Sunday dinner which ends up going into my stomach. I was crushed: we were eating fake and reproduced animals on a daily basis.

Milk seemed so normal since you can pick it up at the grocery store, convenience store, or practically anywhere. But the books I read had me questioning why I would drink milk from a cow if I was not a cow. Cow's milk is used to supply the baby cow with fuel just like a human mother would provide breast milk for her baby. So why was I drinking cow's milk if I'm not a cow? It is no wonder so many new medical conditions and diseases occur in our society. Mankind continually creates new and improved "foods" based on Americans' desires, at the cheapest rate possible, all at the expense of our health.

When I read up on the original "farm to table" practices for most meat in this country and the hard work the body faces once these fake foods enter our body, I knew I had to stop eating meat and cut back on dairy. This led me to find out what other protein alternatives were out on the market and I decided to shape my lifestyle not only healthier but also vegetarian.

The last component in the macronutrient chain is fat. Fat "provides essential fatty acids and is necessary for the proper functioning of cell membranes, skin, and hormones and for the transporting fat-soluble vitamins."[3] I learned that there was saturated and unsaturated fat in the foods we ate, and we should add more unsaturated fats to our diet. Not only should the fat come from unsaturated fats, but the portions of food that contain these fats should be smaller since the energy contained in these foods is so dense. Low-fat diets were commonly advertised around this time and it made sense in theory to me, so I decided to buckle down and cut back on all fatty foods. I kept my fat content low by using cooking spray instead of olive oil and only eating egg whites instead of the yolk, very little nuts and nut butters, and keeping cheese to a minimum. I did not include more fats into my diet until later on in my weight loss journey.

Deciding to eat healthier and becoming vegetarian at the same time was a challenge for me, especially at such a young age as well. For one, becoming vegetarian in the black community, or in the country in general in the early 2000's, was almost completely unheard of. Restaurants in Hampton Roads did not cater to a vegetarian lifestyle; this was no metropolitan city. During this time and in my circles, the Internet was not a popular tool to use, so I had no support groups to turn to for people who became vegetarian. There were no Facebook groups I could log onto, no social media site with motivational quotes saying, "Yeah you can do this." The internet was not abuzz with vegetarian recipes. Nah, it was me all by myself deciding to go this non-meat route, so it was not easy. My family and pretty much everyone I knew was not about this non-meat lifestyle and thought I was crazy and just going through a phase. I remember going into restaurants and explaining I wanted the sides and not the meat and waiters would look at me as if I had 3 heads. Even some restaurants who just had vegetables would season their vegetables with meat, so I was at a loss as well. And some people just did not get it. I remember several times being over at a friend's house and they ordered pepperoni pizza. I said I could not eat that because I was vegetarian, so they were like just take the meat off of it or just eat around it. What?!?!? Clearly, they did not get the memo when I said, "I don't eat meat" means I don't eat meat at all.

I didn't take it to heart that so many people were not supportive because there really was not a substantial frame of reference in society about a vegetarian lifestyle. It was so foreign to our upbringing in this country that I just decided to figure it out on my own as I went along. I researched all of the non-meat protein sources available at that time and tried most of them out. After scouring the internet and what limited information it had, I headed to the grocery store and decided most of my protein sources would come from eggs, nuts, and veggie meat-based products such as veggie burgers, veggie meat balls, veggie sausages, veggie ground crumbles, as well as, beans, protein shakes, and tofu. I still ate cheese but was never a big cheese person so that was not a big staple of my diet. I ate it maybe 1-2 times a week and in small amounts at that. Ice cream made me go to the bathroom within 2 minutes flat so I gave that up way before I was vegetarian. Drinking cow's milk was not a regular occurrence in my diet either since I only had it with cereal, so the transition to soy milk and then eventually to almond milk was easy. But switching from eating chicken for lunch and dinner every day for years was probably my biggest hurdle. I mean, I had to give up General Tso's Chicken, turkey at Thanksgiving, and barbecue chicken at the cookouts, WTF? And no one was forcing me to do this – I came up with this stinking bright idea on my own? Even worse, as I mentioned earlier, Hampton Roads is not a major metropolitan area, so it is not progressive in the sense of culture and dining. To my knowledge, there were not any vegetarian restaurants in the early 2000's in the Tidewater area. My options at restaurants were as such: whatever vegetable side dish they had on the menu (which was usually 3 small stalks of broccoli), salad, or a sandwich in which you asked to keep everything on the sandwich but the meat. Lastly, removing the meat from the sandwich would usually erupt into a 5-minute conversation because the waiter would always think they misheard me and would have difficulty ringing up the order.

Most people would have given up considering some of the difficulty I faced with this new lifestyle. The challenges I faced with eating in restaurants and going to family functions, at a time when being vegetarian was not something easy to abide by, were major. But the truth is, you could not have paid me to eat chicken, turkey, and beef again; it was just too unhealthy of a thing to put daily into my temple, so I adjusted. I started to cook food more often so that I had more control over what was going into my body. I got snobby about what food I ate, what restaurants I visited, and what I did to my body day in and day out. I treated my body as if it was a gift from God that I could not fill with unhealthy things. I mean we only get one body, so I needed to take care of it as such. To this day, most of my meals come from my house instead of a restaurant. What is considered "most?" If we are eating 3 meals a day at 7 days a week, that is 21 meals a week. Out of 21 meals, generally speaking, 1 of my meals a week could come from a restaurant, shop, or cafe. I am not saying I am doing serious cooking every day, it's just a habit for me to physically curate my meals instead of giving that authority to someone else. I'll explain more about how I approach meals in a later chapter.

So once I figured out what macronutrients are and decided that I was going to be vegetarian, the question remained: What is the plan, Tasha? What am I going to eat? How am I going to work out? Mind you, I did not write anything down, I just started winging it. But I was winging it with a WHY? I asked myself WHY am I going to turn my diet upside down? Why am I going to work out several days a week when I could chill instead? My answer was simple: because I wanted to take an active part in living my *best* life. I'd been taking a very sedentary, go with the flow, whatever happens, happens, lifestyle, and I was over it. It was time for a complete overhaul once and for all, and I was ready for the process.

C H A P T E R 5

I WAS FOCUSED ON "THE JOURNEY," NOT THE DESTINATION

FORMATTING A WEIGHT LOSS PLAN

Since I have been a fitness enthusiast for most of my life, I knew I wanted to go for the gusto when it came to the workout portion of getting healthy. It was a no-brainer that I was going to be doing cardiovascular training as a part of my workout routine. The elliptical and I were already a great team, so I was going to keep the party going with that. I loved being active ever since I was young and was up for trying new things, so I knew I wanted to add weight training to my workout routine. I read several articles explaining how incorporating weight training into your fitness routine could help you achieve some awesome results, and that's been true from when I started my research on weight training to now. Evidence suggests "ten weeks of resistance training may increase lean weight by 1.4 kg, increase resting metabolic rate by 7%, and reduce fat weight by 1.8 kg."[1]

---

4   Westcott, WL. Resistance Training is Medicine: Effects of Strength Training on Health. <u>Current Sports Medicine Reports. 2012 Jul-Aug;11(4):209-16.</u>

I did not have a specific look I wanted to achieve by lifting weights, but I knew that since I was in poor shape, my weekly fitness plan would include weight lifting.

Once I realized my workout was going to consist of weight training and cardio, I needed to figure out how to create a workout. You could look at several *Shape* and *Self* magazines for they're monthly workout guide but actually creating a challenging workout day-to-day that works for you could become a challenge. I did not know how to physically train my body to lose weight. Truth is, I did not spend too much time figuring out how to create the perfect workout routine because at this point I was itching just to move again (…*sometimes, the best way to start is just by moving…*). I looked at several magazine articles, watched more fitness workouts on tv, reviewed the VHS workout tapes I used to do back in the day, and created some circuits for all of my main body parts and then headed for a gym.

The gym was also a perfect distraction for the first real job I finally got post-college. I ended up obtaining employment at The Pines. Whenever I would mention to people I used to work at The Pines, about half of the people would say something along the lines of 'Ohhhh I have a cousin who worked there. I have heard its pretty rough.' Well, let me tell you, rough is an understatement. The Pines facility I worked at provided 24-hour supervision to youth who suffered with mental issues so severe that they were considered a threat to themselves and/or the public. The Pines was fortunate enough to hire me as a counselor, but I was unfortunate to be put in a position that was way more than I bargained for. The counselor position, though highly needed to provide care and treatment to a unique group of youth in our community, proved to be highly stressful for me, unrewarding, and did nothing to improve the negative feelings I had about myself. What's even worst? I definitely could not afford a personal trainer as my job working with The Pines only paid $9.36/hr, so I had to wing this weight loss thingamajig myself. None of my friends were into working out and neither was my family. The only person I personally knew who actually worked out was my cousin Kevin, so I asked him about getting me on the military base to workout with him in the gym. Once he got the approval, I latched onto him like the cream in my Oreos.

Kevin had been working out for years on base, so I hopped at the chance to work out with him. He was my only hope in "officially" starting a workout program and I was thankful he got me access. What I did not take into consideration when it came to working out with my cousin was that he was a 6'2 male who was already in shape and lifted heavy weights. I, on the other hand, was an obese woman who was out of shape and could not lift anything but my fork for more lasagna - man, I used to love eating big plates of lasagna. *My Aunt Vee used to make the best meaty and cheesy lasagna in the world.*

Anyway, once we got to the gym, Kevin, like most men, headed to work his chest and shoulders with barbells, weight plates, and curl bars. Everything was just so big and bulky in that section of the gym that I was instantly intimidated. What's worse is 95% of the people in the gym were male, so I really felt that I stood out as an eyesore with my little 5lb weights doing biceps curls for the 48th time, dressed in bulky sweat pants and sweat shirts like people would not recognize that I was overweight. The first gym I attended was a very daunting place, but I started to fall in love with the feel of dominating the weight, rep by rep. I had felt a loss of control in my life, and this dominance over something that was heavy and challenging – something that I could do on a weekly basis – gave me a rush like no other. I loved pushing myself to the limit while doing a leg press. In fact, my legs were the strongest part on my body and I loved lunging and squatting 'til the death of me (now, my clients could, and would, back this statement up). So my fear for the place meant nothing in comparison to the feelings I got after crushing a workout and feeling sore once I finished. A sense of accomplishment rushed over me after I completed each workout. So yeah, I was there for the long-haul.

I took my time in the gym and tried out most of their machines to get a sense of how they felt to my body. Becoming comfortable in the gym allowcd me to curtail a fitness program that usually included me performing 12-20 reps, performing 3-4 sets of each exercise before moving on to the next. Not only did I focus on working the legs, (which I felt was my problem area), but I would also work my shoulders, back, chest, biceps, triceps, and abs. Again, all of these movements and manipulation of these machines initially felt weird and cumbersome, but something inside me just said, "Stick with it, Tasha." As for the intensity of my workouts, I was not trying to die after each workout and I did not want the workout to be easy. I would say I found a sweet spot with my workouts; the weight I lifted was moderately challenging so much so that I was barely able to finish those last 2 reps of each set. It really was not pushed at that time in society for women to lift weights unless you were a body builder, but I remember looking at fitness guru Donna Richardson and ESPN's early morning workout videos that had small, lean women lifting weights right along with the men, just at a smaller weight. I did not want to be as small as them, but I remember thinking, 'hmmm they're muscular but they're still feminine at the same time,' so I pumped that weight, honey.

Once Kevin and I finished our individual strength training, we met back up to do our cardio together. We worked out together an hour or so about 3-4 times a week for months, and I loved it! I will always be grateful to my cousin Kevin for being part of the "jumpstart" to this journey.

LOSING WEIGHT IN THE STONE AGE (NO SOCIAL MEDIA)

I started my fitness journey in the non-social media age and let me tell you; it was a much more difficult time for someone to lose weight than it is now. 15 years ago when I started this journey there was no Myspace, Facebook, Instagram, YouTube, Pinterest, fitness blogs, or online weight-loss group chats. I did not have the 24-hour, 365 days a year access to any and everything that is fitness-related that someone now has if they are trying to lose weight. I did not have the benefit of waking up every morning to see motivational quotes, women that looked like me lifting weights on a regular basis doing various workouts, or all of these before and after weight loss pictures of women on a minute, hourly, or daily basis at the touch of my fingertips. Nah, nope, never happened. Fitness-related tv shows usually aired when I was already at work, so I only saw them if I had to miss work for some reason. Fitness magazines hit shelves once a month and they only featured one workout, and often times they were not challenging enough for what my body was capable of at the time. There was a focus on aerobic-based exercises that really only seemed to help if you were already on the small side. The VHS workout tapes I purchased were challenging, but it was easy to get tired of performing the same exercises every single day.

Weight Watchers meet-ups, Curves circuit work-outs, and Jazzercise fitness classes were popular at the time and I could've made my way there to connect with possibly like-minded individuals. However, to be honest, those companies at the time did not seem appealing to a 23-year-old single, sensitive, black woman like myself. Group members most often could be seen as 45 years old and up Caucasian women, so I really was not jumping at the chance to sign up. These companies weren't necessarily catering to my demographic and I did not feel comfortable joining a group as such. Also, I made an effort for my workout routines to have a major focus on strength training, while most of these programs had more of a focus on calisthenics. Needless to say, I had to become inventive with my workout routines since it was hard to get on-going help in the fitness realm at that time.

In addition to social media not being a "thing" and local fitness companies not being well-suited for me, there was little fitness technology to assist you with creating or tracking your fitness and nutrition plan. Fitbit watches, calorie tracker apps, MyFitnessPal app, healthy recipe websites and apps, and Apple watches were not in existence. To keep track of my routine, I wrote down each week what body parts I would focus on and created a list of all the exercises I knew. I worked from those lists each week and added on additional exercises to the list when I found out about them or created my own exercises. Since fitness apps were not around, I used the Talk-Test to gauge whether my workout was challenging enough. If I was easily able to talk to someone during my workout or after I finished a set of exercises then I was not working hard enough. I would either move faster through my set (while still maintaining proper form), increase the weight, or incorporate a different move to increase the difficulty of the workout. Instead of looking through my favorite nutrition blogger's Instagram feed for meal ideas, I repeatedly looked through my mom's two Betty Crocker cookbooks to figure out ways to cook and "healthify" meal dishes. Basically, I worked with what I had (and did not take time to complain about what I did not have) to make this my best start ever.

Looking back at this time—even though I did not have access to the technology we have now as way to encourage and motivate me to reach my goals—it has made me appreciate that this was truly a self-taught journey. Kevin's willingness to have me tag along with him gave me the self-confidence to push further day after day along this ride. There is nothing like having someone on your side who believes in you, despite the fact that you failed several times before. Thank you, Kevin.

As soon as Kevin and I started working out, I immediately made small changes to my diet and actually stuck with it! I did not wait until l got in a nice, cushiony groove with working out. Wondering why did not I wait? It is simple: I was tired of waiting to live my life. I had been waiting to live my life for *years*. As you might remember, I tried some drastic strategies to lose weight (i.e. starvation, weight loss shakes, weight loss pills, etc.) in the past and failed. I reminded myself that I wanted a life, not a season or two or three years to myself… I wanted a *life*. My weight loss needed to be permanent, so this transition into eating healthier needed to be constant but gradual. I did not want to feel like I was missing out but rather like I was learning to appreciate food in a different way.

KEEP THE FOOD SIMPLE

My initial food strategy was quite simple: I stopped eating fried foods and Lay's Sour Cream and Onion potato chips. That is it, chile. This may not seem like a lot to some people, but this was 80% of my diet growing up. I, like most teenagers, loved fast food! I mean, you could not tell me that the Quarter Pounder with cheese from McDonald's and a large serving of fries was not the best meal on earth. Captain D's two-piece fish dinner with coleslaw and hush puppies was an absolute missile. And last, but most certainly not least, was Chanello's Pizza – a 1-topping pizza with ranch sauce for $5.99 that, with tax, came to $6.59. That was an absolute steal, and for good reason: it was delicious.

French fries from McDonald's, Wendy's, OreIda steak fries, and Captain D's played a weekly role in my life (S/n: Burger King's French fries tasted awful. I would just get a Whopper from Burger King and then drive to McDonalds to get the fries – it was the best of both worlds, baby!). I ate French fries 3-5 times a week because they are magical. Lay's Sour Cream and Onion potato chips were my after-dinner coffee or dessert. As soon as I finished eating the meal that my mother prepared for my sister and I, I would sneak the bag into my room and eat them. Apparently, the potato chips functioned as a palette cleanser or official finish to my meal. I assume they still make them and that someone else in this world understands the herb and salt combination that occurs in this delicacy. I ate chips about 4-5 times a week. The number of calories in fast food and potato chips are so dense that when I replaced these foods with baked chicken, rice and green beans, I immediately lessened the calories I was taking in on a daily basis. I did not replace the chips with a lower-fat snack – I just stopped eating them. I am not saying I never snacked when I started my weight loss journey, but I just knew I was not hungry when I ate the chips, so there was no need to replace them with something else. Since I stopped eating at fast food restaurants, that meant I was not drinking soda anymore. Soda was not a huge factor in my life since I just drank it out of habit because that is what came with the meal. I replaced soda with low sugar juice, like Ocean Spray's Light Cranberry Juice. I also drank more water, but I was not drinking a ton of water like I do now – I just upped my in-take a bit.

Several weeks after I adapted to becoming a healthier-eating vegetarian, I decided to reduce the portion of food I was eating. I had been overeating all my life and

I knew it. It does not take a rocket science to figure out that scooping two cups of spaghetti on your plate is more than you need for a meal. I knew that ladle I was using to scoop my potatoes was putting about a pound of food on my plate and I had not even gotten to my protein. I knew that eating a 12-inch sub from Subway was a problem. We all know when we are being greedy and could scale back on the size of our plate, it's just a matter of doing something about it. This time around I stopped it. Carbohydrates were scaled back to between a 1/2 cup -3/4 cup, no exceptions. I initially measured the food to see how much was in a 1/2 cup and was pissed off when it came to how much rice that amounts to for a meal. I was equally pissed off when it came to cereal. I measured out 3/4 cup of my beloved Captain Crunch cereal and instantly had an attitude. How did they expect me to just eat 3/4 cup of cereal and call this a meal? I kept the smaller portions for rice and spaghetti which were my typical carbs. As far as cereal goes, I just gave up on it. Most cereal had way too much sugar in it anyway, so even choosing the healthier options like as Special K or plain Cheerios was too boring for me. Furthermore, I could not bring myself to eat that small amount of cereal: I just stopped eating it altogether.

So to tie it up in a nut shell, here is what I did to start on my initial (and consistent) weight loss journey: I worked out 4 to 5 times a week with a combination of weight lifting and cardio; I stopped eating fast food and potato chips; I became a vegetarian; I stopped drinking soda and instead drank light juice drinks and water; and I scaled back on my portions of food and instead ate normal portions of food.

DID I EAT ANY CHEAT MEALS?

Well, what about cheat meals, I hear you ask? Desserts? Alcohol? Cheat meals were a no. Desserts were a no. Alcohol was a no. My reason for having no cheats was simple: I had been "cheating" all my life. I made sure to satisfy all of my cravings on a daily and weekly basis and I could feel it. My body felt heavy, bruised and abused from eating whatever I wanted and I was over it. I wanted to know if it was possible for me to feel anything other than "heavy," so I was willing to overhaul whatever I ate in the past and that included cheat meals. So no more spinach dip and tortilla chips, no more greasy Chinese food, no more fried spicy chicken wings, no more chocolate chip pancakes, no more pizza and no more desserts. Alcohol was not a big deal to me in my 20's. I did not start to enjoy the taste of alcohol until I reached about 31 years old, so it played no part in my initial weight loss journey.

What played a big role in my life before I started on this journey was dessert. I was (and still am) an official dessert aficionado. (You'll learn more about my dessert struggles in later chapters.) If there was a certification out here for a dessert specialist, I would have had it. In fact, I could have become the "master" dessert expert and then trained others on how to get to the top of their class. My sweet tooth was sweet as can be. I like my desserts super rich. When others took three bites of chocolate cake with chocolate frosting, topped with chocolate ganache and chocolate chips and said, "Wow that's enough, it's too sweet," I would shrug my shoulders and keep going for the kill. Since I liked to bake (and even considered going into business as a baker earlier in life), I would make brownies, cookies, cakes, and cheesecakes—and then— *more* brownies, cookies, cakes, and cheesecakes, all from scratch. I baked them for others *and* for myself. I was not keen on scaling down a recipe just for one serving, so if I decided to make a personal batch of cookies or brownies, I could easily eat the whole batch and not think twice about it. I had no off-switch: nothing was too sweet for me and no slice was too big for me. So when I decided to give up dessert without hesitation, I knew there was a real change that was occurring within me. I knew that there was a sense of urgency brewing inside of me that wanted to feel something new.

The fast food, chips, and dessert still tasted good – I mean, I did not start hating them just because I was changing my diet. But it was as if my desires for those things diminished. These foods were not feeding me the way I needed to be fed at that point in my life. It did not give me enjoyment or satisfy the craving I had inside of me because *I was craving something that food could not satisfy.* I was craving a look on the other side of the wall. I wanted to know once and for all how it felt to wake up in the morning and not automatically look down at how huge my legs were. I wanted to know what it felt like to be able to fit into all of the clothes in my closet instead of only having one small section of clothes that fit my body. I wanted to know what it felt like to go in a room full of women or men and not feel self-conscious about people staring at how much I weighed. I wanted to feel comfortable walking into a store knowing I could go in the "young women" section and find something to wear instead of heading to the "full-figured" section. Most importantly, I wanted to feel more comfortable about how I looked when I glanced into the mirror. I wanted to feel better about myself to myself so that food would not play the star role in my life anymore; it had to settle for being a supporting cast member. I started to take charge of my day-to-day life and that included ensuring that, "cheat foods" took a backseat.

ANY INITIAL GOAL SETTING?

I did not set out to lose a certain number of pounds or to have a certain waistline size. I just knew that what I'd been doing in the past was not what I wanted to do in the future and that I needed a lifestyle change. I just wanted to feel healthier day in and day out in general, and I hoped that weight loss would become a by-product of that shift.

I got into a groove of going to work, coming home, changing clothes and then meeting up with Kevin to head to base to workout. On the weekends, I would head to Mount Trashmore (a neighborhood park) to walk. I did not meal prep any of my foods as that really was not a "thing" back in the day. There were no meal prep containers and no recipes that explained how to cook healthy meals in bulk for the week. I just knew I needed to eat a lean protein, healthy starch, and vegetable while keeping those portions in check every day. Some of the meals I ate came from my mother (or I just ate the starch and vegetable she prepared) and I prepared my protein or would make my entire meal separate from what my mother cooked. I moved out of my mother's house about a year into my weight loss journey and got an apartment. Once I moved, all of my meals were prepared by myself.

My motto when approaching food today is the same as it was the day I started: keep it simple. I'm a foodie at heart, so I get a kick out of trying to cook different meals to satisfy the variety and love I have for food. But for the love of God, I had to keep my meals simple so I could stick with it. Any meal taking longer than 20 minutes to cook and/or requiring 8-9 or more ingredients was not going to happen. In order for me to stay consistent on the journey, the food part not only had to be healthy, but also easy to whip up. I cooked about 2-3 times a week with leftovers to spare.

Here is the initial approach I used to craft healthy vegetarian meals:

- Breakfast really did not require any cooking since I ate nothing requiring a skillet and a spatula during the week. Examples of food choices were yogurt, fresh fruit, oatmeal, hard boiled eggs, and veggie sausage links.
- For lunch, I mostly ate salads and sandwiches (which is what most people usually eat for lunch whether they are looking to be healthy or not) and an apple, orange, or peach on the side.
- Dinner is what usually required preparation, so I cooked on off-days from the gym, regardless if it fell on a Friday, weekend or not. My meal consisted of one of the vegetarian proteins I spoke of in Chapter 3 and a serving of one starch and a ton of veggies.

Once I ran out of food, I went right back to the grocery store, not the drive-thru, to get more. When I did eat out or went out of town, I always chose the healthiest options they had on the menu because I did not want to mess up my daily routine, the pleasure my body now felt in eating healthy foods, and this new vibe I had running through my spirit. It became a habit for me to feel light on my feet as opposed to lethargic with the 'itis' every Friday, Saturday, and Sunday. I did not make a public declaration to my friends and family that I decided to change my lifestyle, I just woke up one day with this fire to change, so that is what I did.

I got into a smooth groove of working out and eating right, and I was completely fine with it. I wasn't like "oh wow, this is great, I'm a healthy person! I'm the bomb!" Nor, did I feel super skinny once I started working out. I more so felt like I got into a routine of living my life this way and *it became a habit.* I became a person who not only worked a 40-hour-a-week job, brushed my teeth, washed my face, and paid my bills, but who also worked out weekly (no excuses) and made a conscious decision every time I put something in my mouth for it to be a healthy choice. My choices for my life now consisted of me adapting this food and workout regimen into my new lifestyle.

About 2 and a half months into this new lifestyle, I decided to step on the scale in the gym. I don't know why, on this day, I decided to step on the scale this day because as long as I could remember, I despised stepping on the scale. The scale has never been my friend; it has been my enemy and bully for life. As I mentioned before, every single time I've ever gone to the doctor for a check-up, regardless if I was 9 or 19 years old, the scale always went up and it made me feel absolutely horrible inside for the next 2-5 days. After every scale fiasco, I would eat something greasy or sweet to soothe my pain. So needless to say, I was a bit apprehensive of stepping on this time bomb. I mean, what if it said I gained weight? What if my weight stayed the same? That would mean I have been doing all of this no-meat like a weirdo and avoiding Oreo cheesecake all this time for nothing? In the past, I tried different weight loss strategies and failed, so a lot was riding on this moment. As I started to step up on the scale, I felt as if I was running in slow motion through the desert while wearing a sweatsuit towards a scale over the horizon, while praying "please baby Jesus, give me a good sign." I could feel my blood pressure rising in my chest and for a few minutes it felt as if I stopped breathing. As I began to close my eyes, I felt one foot step on to the scale. Then, my other foot landed on the scale. When both feet were firmly planted on the scale, I finally opened my eyes. The scale read that I lost 14 pounds.

To this day, that was one of the most shocking and memorable moments that has ever occurred in my life (and I will never forget it). I stood on the scale perplexed and amazed at what just happened. I kept staring at the numbers to make sure they really were appearing the way my eyes and brains were interpreting them. I actually lost weight! I, Tasha Turnbull, lost 14 pounds. You might think I would have noticed I lost some weight before this moment, but the truth is that I never could tell whether I had lost anything based on how my clothes were fitting because I only felt comfortable wearing oversized clothes like big t-shirts, sweaters, and sweat pants. So this moment was the very first moment where I realized that it was true – I was a person who could change the trajectory of my life. I could change what had been going on in my life for the past 5, 10, 15, 20 years. I had doubted myself all these years and now I saw that I could change how my life was going to look.

TIME TO CELEBRATE?!?

I did not celebrate by baking a cake or eating chips. Are you kidding me? After I just found out that I lost pounds? I was not about to kill that vibe with something that seemed so short-sighted. I had just had a taste of success from the one thing I have failed over and over for the past 23 years and that was all the confirmation I needed that I was on the right track to go for even more. GAME ON!

CHAPTER 6

SELF-TALK, SELF-LOVE

As I LOOKED back over those two and a half months prior to stepping on that scale, I knew there was something different going on inside of me. I noticed that I started to talk to myself in an encouraging kind of way. Usually, my self-talk would consist of me making sure I did a good job at work and school, keeping up with paying my bills on time, and checking in with friends. I had the same weekly routine that I'd been following for years, but I never really talked to myself about *me*, you know? I never talked badly to myself, but because I did not like what I looked like, I neglected myself. I was afraid to face what was going on with my body and my emotions, so I moved my emotions and feelings to the back of the bus. I ugly-ducklinged myself, all by myself. As I got older, I did not need the teasing from the kids in elementary school and middle school as I became my own worst enemy. Those bottled up feelings led to the depression that came to a head once I finished college.

But once I started "The Journey" this time around, that changed. Instead, I talked to myself about how I was going to maneuver throughout each day. It was as if my feelings and emotions now had somewhere to go. They weren't just laying around in my head causing stress, back pain, weight gain, and emotional turmoil, they were put to work to take away the mental pain I was feeling inside. My being was crying out, craving a different type of routine, order, and stability, and that is exactly what I created for myself. At the beginning of each week, I planned out what 4 days I was going to work out that week, and I stuck to it. I talked to myself about what I was going to eat for the day, and that is what I ate.

When I started to follow what I set out for myself, it gave me self-confidence. I did not care what was going on outside and around me. This new workout/eat right thing was giving me all kinds of energy and life, and I was not gonna stop this train for anything or anybody. So if I had a doctor's appointment at my regular workout time, I'd switch my workout to later in the evening even if that meant I would get home really late (and I still had to be at work the next day by 7am). Once it was planned, the workout was going to get done by any means necessary. If I was going out with friends, I'd stick with eating a salad. There were not a whole lot of healthy options at most restaurants 15 years ago, other than salads, so that is exactly what I got. I was not mad that I always ate a salad, though; I'd come to love salads, and still do to this day. So I ate my meal with people eating their burgers and fries in front of me and did not care a bit. Now, sometimes I would salivate and stare at their food until they finished that last French fry on their plate, but I just could not bring myself to indulge. I'd come way too far to stop over 10 friggin' French fries. Nope! I stayed on-trend and before you knew it, both our meals were finished and I drove home not feeling depressed about committing the ultimate sin for me: starting over in the morning.

Staying steadfast over the course of those few months gave me a new-found respect for myself. I do not think fitness is the only way people can increase their self-worth, but sticking to this routine day in and day out was something that I've been wanting to achieve for so long. Getting the extra weight off of my body was something that had been holding me down, so when I devised my plan and I started to stick to it, it increased my belief in myself to reach this goal. I was nowhere near losing 100 pounds when I saw the numbers on the scale drop by 14 pounds; however, I was able to accept where I was, and that allowed me to stop judging myself and get on with establishing a healthier routine.

HOW DID I BECOME SO JUDGEY?

Judgement is the main reason why I failed 597 times in the past. I was not bullied in high school and college, probably because I was too busy criticizing myself every single day. And while personal pan pizzas from Pizza Hut and the waffle fries from Chic-Fil-A tasted amazing, I was so disappointed that I was not doing anything to stop myself from eating this way and not fitting most of my clothes. I knew that these foods were causing me to gain weight. Instead of doing something about it, I just sat there with the food judging myself. I felt like such a failure because I was not a small person. Some people wish they had more money, a better job, a cuter wardrobe, or a betting living situation – I just wanted my thighs to not cause a fire storm from walking since they rubbed together all day long. I compared my arms and legs to every single person that I met, and by careful research, deductive reasoning, and several case studies *I knew* had the biggest arms and legs in Hampton Roads. Period. It was so true and you could not tell me otherwise, chile. Some people who have large extremities can move about by walking or jogging and their fat would not move. But my arms and legs would jiggle to no end and it was embarrassing. That's why you could not find me wearing anything fitted in high school and college – I needed to hide that jiggle from everyone else *and* myself. Since I was obsessed with arms and legs, in my mind I characterized people who have small arms and legs as good people and people who have big arms and legs as not so good. Unfortunately, I applied that narrative to myself and felt like such a bad person.

Once Kevin and I got into this routine of working out and I started making small changes with my diet, I found that I had less time to judge how I looked in the moment. A paradigm shift was occurring with what I obsessed over on a daily basis. The effort, time, and energy I previously used to judge and criticize myself transferred to the prepping, planning, and action that I needed to carry out my new lifestyle.

You might think that I am only speaking metaphorically when it comes to this transfer of energy. But how many of you all know what it feels like to be weighed down by the thoughts that swirl around and around in your head? How many times have you said to yourself, "I don't understand why I keep eating these foods every day and then get mad at myself afterwards?" The cycle of eating crap and then being down on yourself has been in effect for so many years that now you are almost conditioned to feel this way regardless of whether you have eaten anything "bad" or not. It could be 7:22am in the morning and you are just mad at yourself for no reason. Mad and stressed the hells bells out by thoughts solely coming from your head and no one else has even talked to you that day. You get tired and then sick and tired of feeling the same way over and over again. Your blood pressure starts to go up when you go to the doctor because you're worried over your weight or the stress of your weight or a combination of the two. Once you start doing this several times a day for years, it starts to take a toll on your mind and body. According to an article published by Suzanne

Segerstrom in the <u>National Center for Biotechnology Information</u>, our immune system is considered an energetically costly immune system and stress plays a role in whether or not our immune system stays balanced.[5] Stress and negative thoughts require a lot of use out of our body which can affect our thoughts, feelings, physical body, and behavior. My whole being was focused on judging myself to no end. So when I started to transfer some of that energy into a productive line of self-talk and self-love, I started to feel lighter. Day by day, I found myself less critical about how I looked and more focused on where I was headed. Yessss, Tasha! I did not feel like I weighed less, but I started to feel this emotional weight come off my shoulders. Once I lessened the self-criticism and head trash, I was able to focus on establishing a plan and habit of action. These habits could only occur once I embraced acceptance and was less judgmental.

ACCEPTANCE ENABLED ME TO BREATHE

There was an acceptance of who I was when I started this "health kick." My thighs still rubbed together and my arms still took up too much land mass, but there was no use in harping on it, you know? I just needed to

---

5 Sergerstrom, S. et. al. Psychological Stress and the Human Immune System: A Meta-Analytic Study of 30 Years of Inquiry. <u>Psychological Bulletin</u>, American Psychology Association. July 2004. Vol. 130. 601-630.

see if this new routine could give me something better than the present. To change my current situation, I had to accept that this *was* my current situation. You cannot change something that you do not think is real or something that you decline to accept. In real life, I was an obese young woman and if I was going to change any of that then I had to realize that it was going to take more than 2 and a half months of training and healthy food to undo what had been going on for years. If I started out as a smaller person trying to lose weight, then maybe all I would've needed was 2 to 3 months to get myself in check. The reality was that I was not a small person. I wore a size 18, my blood pressure was elevated, and I was too tired for someone so young. I did not like what I saw, and I realized that I needed to face myself in the mirror and acknowledge that this is me. Once you accept that, you can focus on improvement and correction.

I did not obsess about reaching a certain size or having definition in my abs, I just wanted to improve the body that God gave me. I didn't put an abnormal amount of pressure on myself to be a size 10 by December. I did not weigh myself each day to see if I lost a pound or not. And I did not want to look like a certain celebrity or fitness personality. When you put an abnormal amount of pressure on yourself to change, it can feel like you are in constant battle with yourself as opposed to playing on the same team. I knew what pressure from within felt like and I did not want any negative self-pressure along this journey. So I did not put any stringent goals on myself. Since I was focusing on building a better me on my own terms and not someone else's, I started to find comfort in being me. I found a routine I liked, lost a few pounds, and was really starting to like working out, so myself and I became cool. I started to encourage myself to try new vegetables, cook new meals, and up the weight I was lifting in my workouts. I was trying so many new things in my life that it was exciting. My lifestyle was changing right before my eyes and I started to feel better about myself and the body that God gave me.

I knew I had the beginnings of self-love when the tone of the words I spoke to myself came from an encouraging and direction-based perspective. I've always been an internally motivated person. Ever since I can remember, I was internally motivated to get good grades in school and to excel in sports. I had perfect attendance throughout elementary school, middle school, high school, and college. I never missed class, ever. I was always on the honor roll and got a thrill out of the teacher calling my name for getting A's and B's each semester. Man, I used to love the bumper stickers we got in elementary school saying that your child was on the honor roll at Coleman Place Elementary; ugh, I lived for that (even though I was not driving a thing). Although my parents could not afford to put me on a recreational sports team to develop my playing skills, I gave my all while performing gymnastics in middle school and playing soccer and basketball in high school. I showed up to practice on time, went through all the drills as best as I could and gave 100% during games. My parents never had to talk with me like, "In this household, we only accept A's and you must abide by the rules." I never felt pressure to become a doctor, a lawyer, or to get straight A's. Honestly, it was not even necessary for them to put pressure on me. I was self-motivated to do a good job at all times. I remember my therapist, years later, asking me why I put so much pressure on myself to be a perfect person if it did not come from my parents. The answer is that I have no idea. All I know is that when I put my mind to something, whether it be positive or negative, I was going to follow through. So once I decided that I was going to take this healthy living project head on, I was all the way in. I am not a gray area type of person, it does not suit me well. If I am out, I'm out. But if I am in, then I am going to see this journey to the end.

According to a study conducted by Janet Buckworth on motivation, "external motivation such as losing 20lbs for your cruise in June, fitting into a sexy dress by your 35th birthday, or obtaining a 28-inch waist by your wedding day can only motivate you for a short period of time. In order to maintain the necessary order and commitment that one needs to stay active enough to lose the weight, the motivation needs to come from within. "[6] I had no pre-set goals about how much weight I wanted to lose or what I wanted my body to look like once I "finished" this journey; those thoughts never crossed my mind. I was not focused on the destination, but on "The Journey." How to live, how to be, and how to maneuver day in and day out along the journey itself, was what fueled my thoughts day to day. To do all of these things, I had to feel like I was the most important person on the planet. I had to love myself enough to want better than what I have achieved in the past (despite past failures) or what I can physically see from far up ahead. Once I got comfortable with being on the journey for a better life, I started to find comfort in looking to myself for support not critique. Increasing my self-love also increased the daily motivation within me to win, excuses were no longer in my vocabulary. Instead of harping on the fact that 82% of the menu at restaurants did not serve healthy food, I found myself making alternative plans, having back up options, and eating small meals before or after I went out in order to make up a full meal. I literally became the work around queen, chile! I did not look at the jar as half empty but half full. Once I started to help myself out as opposed to getting in my own way, I knew I was Team Tasha. I found purpose and a love for myself like no other and it was an awesome feeling.

---

6 Buckworth, J. Lee, R. Regan, G. Schneider, L. DiClemente, C. Intrinsic and Extrinsic Motivation for Exercise: Application to stages of Motivational Readiness, <u>Psychology of Sport and Exercise</u>. 2007. 447-461.

HOW DID I STAY ENCOURAGED?

Staying Encouraged on The Journey

Determined once and for all to follow-through with the healthy lifestyle plan I created, I followed along this path for months. Within the first 12 months, I lost about 50 pounds. Now some of you might be thinking, 'you changed your life for 12 whole months and you only lost 50lbs?'... but I felt like this weight loss was substantial because I did not think it was possible for my body to be anything but big. People in those infomercials with the before and after pictures, losing 18lbs in 3 weeks, were not real humans as far as I was concerned. So the fact that I lost 50 pounds was a freakin' achievement: I felt as if I won $242,000. Although I lost the weight, I did not immediately transition into wearing tube tops, booty shorts and bikinis year-round. My mind did not catch up to the fact that I lost weight at the rate which my body did. I've spoken to other people who have lost a significant amount of weight and they also mentioned that they were still concerned about putting back on the weight so they kept their "big girl clothes." I kept my big girl clothes for years. Shoot, if I looked in my closet now, I know I probably still have a pair of size 14 jeans that I never donated to Goodwill. Nevertheless, the fear of gaining weight did not stop the excitement of pushing through to the unknown. Over the course of the year thereafter, I lost about an additional 25 pounds. So in two years, I lost about 75 pounds.

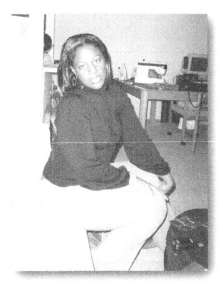

(These are the pictures you take when you start feeling yourself!)

When I decided to write this book, I asked friends and clients what questions they would like to see answered. I also have some common questions that people always ask me about "The Journey" when they first meet me. The top question I always receive is "How did you stay encouraged?" or "Tasha(or what most people call me "T2"), how did you stay committed for so long?" I don't have a short response to that question because there are many factors that are involved with how I got from being an overweight teenager to a woman with definition on her arms, abs, and legs. If you would have told me at 17 years old that I would look the way I do now in my 30's, I would've laughed at you. I could not even begin to conceive that I could be smaller than a size 18. *Puh-lease*. I learned on this journey that you never know how far your body or your mind will take you until you believe in your abilities to stay committed.

I would say there are 3 main things that helped me remain encouraged during this journey. One of them has to do with the fact that I have a mild case of self-diagnosed obsessive-compulsive disorder. Now, I would not say this is a clinical diagnosis because my fixation on "The Journey" did not interfere with me completing non-fitness-related day-to-day activities. But this OCD afforded me the main reason why I was able to stay focused on this journey: it got me "In the zone." Some of my clients have heard me use this term, "In the zone" from time to time. Honey, I was in the zone from the first moment I stepped foot in that gym on base with Kevin. When you are in the zone, you will make a way out of no way because all you see is the finish line. I had tunnel-vision kind of like when you get a new boyfriend. When that new boo hits the scene, it does not even matter if all your friends think he's ugly, in your mind, he is the finest thang on this planet and you would not even see another attractive guy if he walked right up to you (except for Idris Elba, of course). I became fixated on defeating "The Journey" that had beaten me up and crushed my spirit for so many years. I was broken and I found a way to fix myself, so I never let my tools leave my hands: I carried them with me at all times.

One usually does not start off in the zone; it varies from person to person where just the right amount of focus, obsession, adrenaline, fervor, and discipline get flowing through your veins so that you become unstoppable. You are so far gone that no person, object, job, spouse, child, or professor can prevent you from falling off the wagon. You may not be in the pros but you start to operate as an athlete. You recognize the body is the tool you need to win the medal or the championship, so you do everything in your power to optimize the performance of your body to win. Feeling like an athlete, you get comfortable with doing whatever it takes for you to win, be it something you work on monthly, weekly, daily, and/or hourly. When it does not matter how hard or how long it takes you to win because you are that focused on winning, that is when you know you're in the zone.

IN THE ZONE

If Tuesday was my day to work out, then I was going to work out. It didn't matter if I had to stay late at work, after being pissed off by my supervisor, then had to sit in a traffic accident for an additional 45 minutes while in a torrential downpour, I was still going to the gym to hit the weights. It didn't matter if a friend asked me at the last minute to go out to dinner with her to Olive Garden (and those breadsticks used to be the bomb back in the day), I was not going. A guy could've hit me up to go to Red Lobster (...those cheddar bay biscuits...) and I would have passed because Tuesday was my day to work-out. I could've been tired, sleepy, exhausted, sluggish, feeling blah, been on my period, had to find $652.00 to get my car fixed, or just had the worst day in the world... and I still would make it to the gym. The thought of skipping a workout never crossed my mind because it simply was not an option I gave myself. If something happened and I could not make it to the gym (which was a very rare occurrence), I would do a workout video at home. (I had a ton of videos on VHS and you best believe I would work out until my sweat level matched what I got in the gym.) If you allow yourself the option to pass, the thought could start to creep into your mind more often and you could possibly default to that choice. You could end up skipping a workout maybe once a week or once a month. For some people, skipping one or two workouts causes a domino effect for them to skip even more. So for me, I never allowed myself the option; therefore, I never used it. When you're in the zone, how you feel has absolutely nothing to do with how you act; the two are mutually exclusive. I was obsessed with sticking to the plan and moving another day further along on "The Journey." I was able to separate my feelings from the actions I needed to complete to reach my goals, and that is the number one reason how I stayed so long on this journey.

PLAN AHEAD

The second component I used to help me stay encouraged on this journey was my obsession with planning. At this time, I was enthralled with being active, but my knack for planning has always been a part of the narrative from day one. I was a planning aficionado. I loved when the start of school rolled around and I could get a new planner. Ever since I was a kid, I would plan out my school assignments, volunteer activities, tests, and doctor's appointments in my planner. When the summer came around, I still looked in my planner to see what I had planned during the previous school year, and to this day, I have no idea why. Along a similar line, I've always loved looking at recipes and planning out meals (even though in the past they were usually unhealthy meals), seeing how a meal came together one ingredient at time. I took that same love for planning from my school work and baking brownies and put it into planning out my healthy meals, workout days and exercises. There is something about manually writing out your plans for the week in a planner (as opposed to just reciting in my head what I planned to do) that helped me stick to them as well. Gail Matthews, a clinical psychology professor at Dominicana University of California, completed a study that agrees with the idea that people who wrote their goals accomplished significantly more than those who did not write down their goals. [7] I wasn't concerned with writing out what weight loss goals I wanted to achieve, but I was keenly aware of the impact that written planning would have on my focus about what I needed to do when I got to the gym and what I was going to eat from week to week.

Before I started on "The Journey," my Sundays would go like this: I would go to church with my family, eat Sunday dinner early in the day, immediately eat my beloved Lay's Sour Cream and Onion potato chips, watch movies all day, and then bake a cake, cookies, or brownies in the evening. Once I switched, Sundays became my ultimate planning day. How well I planned on Sunday (meaning how much effort I put into planning) would be the main indicator on how well I stuck to my goals for the week. I would plan out what days I would work out and what days I would rest.

---

7 Matthews, G. Strategies for Achieving Goals, Resolutions. Goals Research Summary. May 2015 at the Ninth Annual International Conference of the Psychology Research Unit of Athens Institute for Education and Research (ATINER). http://www.dominican.edu/academics/lae/undergraduate-programs/psych/faculty/assets-gail-matthews/researchsummary2.pdf

During the early stages of my journey, I worked out 4 days a week. I decided to perform cardio on all 4 days and switch up what body parts I wanted to work on those 4 days. I worked legs twice a week because that was my "problem area," and then on the other two days, I would switch up between working biceps, triceps, shoulders, chest and back. As for my abdominal area, I worked it 4 days a week as well. As far as I was concerned, cardio and abs went together, so before I did my cardio I would work on my abs for about 5-10 minutes. I did not want to take a chance and do abs afterwards because I would end up skipping it. My cardio usually consisted of going on the elliptical, me and that thing were BFFS. I loved the elliptical… to me, it was one of the greatest inventions ever.

Meal planning was not a "thing" back in the day. Although Tupperware has been around for decades, people were not prepping meals like grilled chicken, brown rice, and broccoli for 5 days in the early 2000's. To make sure I stuck to my guns with the food, which was way harder to do than it was to stick with the workouts, I would mentally decide what I was going to eat for the week. After church, I went to the grocery to purchase any of the items I needed. I stuck to maybe 2 or 3 different breakfast items, salads that I prepped at home and brought to work, and 2 to 3 different meals for dinner. Breakfast was my favorite meal of the day and it was quite easy for me to make a veggie sausage and fried egg sandwich. I loved making salads for lunch or dinner: they were quick, did not require any cooking, and I could switch up my vegetables and dressings each week to add variety to them. For dinner, I loved stir-fried veggies and tofu over rice, spaghetti with veggie protein, veggie tacos, veggie burgers, and healthy bean burritos. Each week I switched up which 3 vegetables I would eat for the week and made an effort to learn different ways to prepare them.

How did I keep the variety in meals? Any meal that I loved to eat when I went to a restaurant, I basically researched in cooking magazines on how to make a healthier version of it at home. I noticed that the more I loved how my food tasted at home, the easier it became for me to stay consistent. I also want to mention that I've always been a fiscally conservative person. If I did not like some of the trendy health foods on the market, then I was not going to spend my money on it just because it was healthy. I only purchased food I knew I was going to eat. Once these items hit my shopping cart and I purchased them, you better believe I was going to cook and eat them, no excuses. I made an effort not to purchase junk food because, once again, if it hit my shopping cart and I purchased it, I was going to eat it. I was not one of those people who could bring sweets in the house, eat two cookies and then return to what I was previously doing. Nah, to truly feel satisfied I would need to eat the entire pack of cookies. So those items never made into the shopping cart unless I was intentionally having a treat.

The more effort I put into planning out leg exercises to do on Wednesdays and what new spice and vegetable combination I was going to try out for Thursday's dinner, the more reassurance I had that I could live a healthier lifestyle on a permanent basis. I could not wing it day to day on what I was going to eat or else I would have failed. I could not wait until I got to the gym to decide what I was going to do, that would have caused me to just do cardio for 45 minutes and leave. Initially, starting off on this weight loss journey was something similar to me being a baby and a parent, all-in-one. The baby side of me had to step out there and try new meals, new work-outs and still function in the world, while the parent side of me had to remove all the hard corners from the house so I would not bump into them (remove the junk food from the house, plan out my meals ahead of time, stay away from unhealthy restaurants, etc.) This life I was creating for myself felt like a whole new world to me, and I was happily fine with taking the necessary steps to grow. Another way to look at planning for weight loss success could be its comparison to chess (and I'm a chess player). When you are playing chess, it's as if you have to be three steps ahead of your opponent in order to get that check-mate. You could not wait until it was your turn and *then* decide what you were going to do. No, you had to plan, strategize, and charge forward just to make it safely to the next round. The variety I needed (and made sure to create) in my workouts and in my meal options to stay consistent on "The Journey" required strategic planning and I embraced this challenge without complaints. The unwavering effort and attitude with how I approached my planning is one of the reasons why I was able to stick with this change in my lifestyle during those pivotal first 6 months.

ZERO PRESSURE

The third way I was able to stay encouraged on this journey was a lack of pressure. I bolted out of the gates on my race horse ready to get started and finally stick to "The Journey." But the reason why I was able to lose weight and maintain my weight loss over a decade was because I stopped being so hard on myself. As I mentioned before, it was routine for me to see someone slim and automatically start comparing myself to them. I was quite used to being hard on myself about how my legs looked, how my nose looked, how my arms looked, how my thighs jiggled, and even sometimes about the hue of my complexion. I stopped looking back on how many times I failed over the years or how I currently looked. I allowed myself to breathe again, and breathed big, huge breaths. I did not judge myself for only being able to lift 6lbs when doing bicep curls. I just recognized that this was my starting point and then proceeded to move forward.

I've always considered myself a goal-oriented person, meaning that I always structured my life around achieving goals so I knew what I was supposed to be working towards at all times. I knew that if I got A's and B's in high school, and then I would be able to get into a good college with scholarships and grants in my favor. So I made sure I was on the honor roll every single semester while I was in grade school and in high school. I really wanted a car (a Ford Escort, to be exact) while I was in my 2nd year of college, so I got a job working part-time at A&N. I found a used car in the newspaper for $7,000. Given the number of hours I was working, I calculated how many months I would need to work to purchase the car. I made sure I did not spend a dime on frivolous stuff so that I could save up enough money to get a car in order to work even more hours at the store and keep some spending money in my pocket. I was determined.

Setting goals has always helped me stay on target with what I aspired to achieve in life. But when it came time to drop these pounds once and for all, I took a no-goals approach. I did not say to myself that I needed to lose 40 pounds in 6 months or that I needed to drop 10 pounds in 30 days. I did not want the pressure of feeling bad if I did not reach that goal in a specified time. I was swimming in unchartered territory. For the first time in my life, I knew what it felt like to walk out of my house feeling positive about myself. I could go to the store and try on a pair of jeans and know they were going to fit, or maybe I'd even go down a size (MAJOR!). I was feeling more comfortable in my clothes and in my skin, and I did not want to stop this feeling by putting added pressure on my day-to-day routine. I did not weigh myself on a weekly or monthly basis either. If I stepped on the scale and it did not sway in my favor, I did not need the self-ridicule and punishment I would inevitably put myself through. The scale always caused me anxiety so I hardly went on it; I wanted this process to feel as relaxed as possible. Remember, the main reason why I started on this journey was because I felt that I was not participating in my life. I was not looking for a short-term fix, stint, or special project. I wanted to be an active participant in my life and make this lifestyle a permanent fixture… the weight loss was just the icing on the cake.

Because the weight was not the focus, I ended up losing 100 lbs. Had I kept adding on goal after goal after goal in the beginning of the journey, I would have gotten discouraged and fell right on off the wagon. Instead, I maneuvered my way in to the zone, devised a strategy on how I was going to fit this healthier lifestyle into my routine and did not put any unwanted pressure on my spirit as to what would be the result of this new way of living.

CHAPTER 8

WORK/LIFE BALANCE

BUSY AS CRAP BUT STILL LOSING WEIGHT

THE NEXT FEW years of my life consisted of trying to balance my new weight loss with everything else going on. Once I finished undergrad with a degree in Economics and a degree in African and African American Studies, I knew I wanted to be what is called a social entrepreneur. I've always been intrigued with business and producing a product or service that I called my own while helping to make positive changes within peoples' lives at the same time. Upon furthering my knowledge in college about the difficulties facing African Americans in our country—from slavery, to Emancipation, Reconstruction, to the Civil Rights era, the infiltration of drugs in the black community, etc—I recognized that these unfortunate experiences in our history were still having a substantial impact on men, women, and children in the Black community every single day. I knew I wanted to see what I could do to improve the quality of lives of African American men and women in our country and still start up my business; I just did not know in what capacity I was able to achieve both of those goals.

During the time I lost the 75 pounds, I completed graduate school at Old Dominion University with a master's degree in Public Administration. I felt that if I got a degree in Public Administration, I could get a job affecting policy in the country which could help to bring about more equality to minorities such as African Americans. Once I finished my degree, I ended up working a job with the state of Virginia's Disability Services Agency. I also ended up buying a townhouse, moving from Norfolk to Virginia Beach. By the time I graduated from school, the country was in a recession and the housing bubble burst not too long after I purchased my townhouse. To keep up with bills and maintain some disposable income, I worked part-time at Bed, Bath, and Beyond for 2 years.

My state job had me working from 7:00am to 3:30pm, Monday through Friday. I worked 3 times a week at Bed, Bath, and Beyond and the store closed at 10pm on weeknights, so on those days I could not work out. At that time, you could not have paid me to get out of my bed and do a quick 5am workout before heading to work at 7am, so I only worked out in the evening. That left me with 4 days out of the week to get in a workout.

Once I got the part-time job, I had to be even more strategic with meal prepping. I had to bring two meals for me to eat (lunch and dinner) instead of just lunch. I had to work out on the weekends. I really had to make sure I got restful sleep. I noticed if I stayed up late I would have difficulty focusing throughout the day at work, which would affect my decision-making skills in terms of food, so I carried my butt to bed as soon as I got home. I got up about 10 minutes earlier than usual to prep my salads and dinner since I knew I was not doing it the night before. If I was not scheduled to work on Sundays, I made sure to attend church with my mom and grandma because I knew for sure that Sunday was a day and time I could see my family. Even if I had to work on Sunday, sometimes I would go to early service so I could get in some time with the Lord before spending the day at Bed, Bath, and Beyond. My family would always make an effort to get together to celebrate each other's birthdays, so even though I picked up the second job, I made sure I got off in time to attend family functions (or asked fellow employees to switch schedules with me so that I could keep up with all the action). At this time, most of my family knew I was vegetarian and they began to ask me questions on why I started living this lifestyle. I began to explain the importance of adding more vegetables to your diet and what it was doing to improve my health. So slowly but surely, more vegetables (meaning non-starchy vegetables) were making their way onto the food spread to accommodate me (and them as well) at family dinners. I absolutely loved them for it. But the truth is, even if they only served fried chicken and 14 starches for Sunday dinner, it still would not have stopped me from becoming a healthy vegetarian. I started on this journey by myself and could not be mad if other people were not gonna hop on with me; I did this for me and no-one else.

Once the second job was added to my routine, I made sure to take the time to listen to my body. I needed to find out what would help me succeed given that I was using energy for something else (making additional money) unrelated to weight loss. I knew I needed sleep. I was never a #teamnosleep type of person, and no one else should be either. It has been said that getting less than 6 hours of sleep can cause weight gain, decreases your ability to fight food cravings once you wake up, can increase your caloric intake, and can decrease your metabolism.[8] I needed all-hands on deck in order to continue to lose weight and maintain my weight loss, so I made sure to get my sleep.

I really did not have a booming social life prior to losing weight *or* after losing weight, so I was not focused on keeping up with the Joneses. I have always had friends and we would communicate daily, weekly or monthly, but I never felt the desire to always be out every weekend. Don't get me wrong, I liked to hang out, break it down on the dance floor whenever the DJ plays my song, and try out new restaurants, but I also was a homebody. I loved

---

8 Benedict, C. Acute Sleep Deprivation Enhances the Brain's Response to Hedonic Food Stimuli. Journal of Endocrinology and Metabolism. 2012 Mar; 97(3) :E443-447.

spending time at my little townhouse and just chilling under my favorite throw. I have never felt threatened by people who had more money than me so I also was not in competition with anyone else. I did not need to have all the latest clothes, shoes, or bags. I just wanted to feel better about my own dag-on life. Men have always been pretty sporadic in my life so they were not really a factor when I was knee-deep into my weight loss journey. Although a hardcore breakup with a boyfriend that resulted with me slashing some tires and providing me the fuel to work out would have given some juicy drama to this book, it just would not be true. I did not have kids throughout "The Journey," so that did not play a role in occupying my time, effort, or money. Since I got school out of the way, the major issues I had to deal with were my two jobs keeping me busy and keeping my mental health in order to accept and maintain this weight loss. And, to be honest, that was more than enough for me.

By focusing on living a better life on my own terms, I was better able to prioritize this healthy lifestyle at the top of my to-do list. It was completely ingrained in my mind that I was now a healthy person and my thought patterns reflected this line of thinking day after day. I could not fathom the thought of "starting over on Monday." So instead of eating out with my friends, sometimes I would eat before I arrived and just have something to drink at the restaurant. I turned out to be a pretty decent cook, so I'd catch up with friends by inviting them over for a healthy vegetarian meal I wanted to try out or to taste my homemade sweet potato pancakes I made for Sunday brunch. Instead of sitting on the couch with nothing to do on the weekends, I would take my butt to the gym for an extra workout, even if it was only for 30 minutes. I stopped circling around the parking lot trying to find a spot close to the store and I stopped taking the elevator at work. I did not tell myself, "Tasha, you MUST eat healthy or use must get up and go to the gym." It became a habit of mine to be active; no one pushed me to do these things, it just came naturally because my body got used to being active on a regular basis and not feeling lazy and lethargic after finishing a meal.

Feeling accustomed to being light on my feet also played a role in how I approached cheat meals back in to my life. I decided to permanently stay out of restaurants where I knew I would suffer utter damage to my goals. In the early 2000's, certain franchise restaurants and myself had to part ways because I was so emotionally involved in their food. I gave up Olive Garden because the breadsticks and dipping sauce were a problem. I was a dipping professional. The blondie from Applebee's was a missile. And my recovery time from eating at Cold Stone Creamery was just too severe to chance it ever again. I loved Cold Stone Creamery to death, but the ice cream, cookie dough, chocolate chips, and waffle cone topped with the chocolate sauce and caramel sauce was too much for me to handle like I did in the past. So I declined. I decided to give up these meals because it would start a domino effect in me wanting something else sweet the next day and the next day, so I backed off. I had to be two steps ahead of myself to make sure I did not fall off track, you know? To keep myself sane, my "cheat treats" were smaller in size and fewer in between. I did not set out each week which day I was going to have a "cheat meal," I would more so assess where I was at mentally with my relationship with food at the time (eating intuitively).

If I was feeling like I was struggling a bit with overeating healthy foods, not pushing myself 100% in my workouts, or mad that a guy I was dating at the time was not acting right, I would not allow myself the "cheat." The only times I would allow myself (or feel comfortable) to cheat is if I was in a good groove with my relationship with food. I took this stance on cheat meals because I noticed that when I was in a good relationship with food, I could enjoy the "cheat" and then return to my normal, healthy eating habits. If I used the cheat for anything other than the enjoyment of food, I knew I would not be satisfied and would subsequently move on to eating other junk food. Once I started to research what is in the food we eat, I found out that sugar is addictive. Since I have an addictive personality and I like sweets, and sugar was known to be addictive, this trio could easily result in an epic downfall of monstrous proportions (even to this day). So I had to restrict myself on the sweets if I wanted to maintain my weight and talk myself off the ledge hundreds of times to make sure I was eating desserts for the right reasons. On average, I'd say I was eating a "cheat meal/dessert" maybe 2 to 3 times a month. I did not feel like I was missing out because I was still able to enjoy my desserts, hang out with friends, and remain steadfast along "The Journey." Having a few cheats a couple of times of month kept me balanced, kept my cravings in-check, and kept my feet permanently planted along the right path.

My life was not chaotic, but it was busy from all of the hours I was working at both jobs, my workouts, the meal prepping, and thinking of my next move. But prior to getting started on this healthy lifestyle, however, I had always been someone that was in my own head worrying, thinking, and obsessing over everything and nothing. Being an internally motivated person also meant that I was always thinking about getting over that next hurdle in life; I never slowed down. Because I was so driven I experienced difficulty with learning to relax. Studies have shown that working out can help to relieve stress, calm your nerves, and help you to feel a release once those endorphins started to rush through your body.[9] Well, when I worked out, I did not feel less stressed. I would use my workout time to work through decisions I

---

9 Seaward, BL. Physical Exercise: Flushing Out The Stress Hormones. <u>Essentials of Managing Stress</u>. 3rd Edition. Jones and Bartlett Publishers. 2014.

needed to make in life or plan out the next task I needed to do once I left the gym. Workouts became habitual and a means to end, but it was not a stress-reliever.

My mood still fluctuated up and down like it did in the past. I was trying to work through several things running around in my head such as learning to embrace the weight loss, seeing myself for who I currently am, trying to appreciate life for what it is and live in the moment, working through family issues, and dealing with the fact that guys are crazy and none of the men I met seemed to have their life together and were only interested in dating 22 women at the same time. I stopped going to therapy years ago, but I decided to go back because my mood would stay too low for too long. I was right back to feeling like that Cymbalta commercial. I knew I was not feeling like myself, so I decided to resume therapy and ended up going for several years. I needed an ear to help me sort through all of the issues constantly running through my head. I had my mom and friends whom I would talk to about these issues, of course, but I felt like I needed a 3rd party to help me make sense of why I kept obsessing over the same things over and over and over again.

By incorporating therapy back into my life, little by little, it helped me to think more clearly about where I was in time. I stopped worrying so much about the future and focused on what I could do to enjoy the fruits of my labor and all that the Lord has given me thus far in life. The clarity provided from therapy, along with my drive as an internally motivated person, helped me to be a better decision-maker concerning work, eating healthy, working out, and speaking up more for myself. I stopped hanging around people who only ate junk food or always had something negative to say or who would joke about me always eating healthy food. I know for some people, it can make them nervous when you are not following the crowd and decide to do your own thing, but I could not worry about them. Shoot, I'm still trying to hold my own self up above water. I also stopped responding back to guys who were only interested in texting and meeting up with me after 10pm. Under previous circumstances, I would have still entertained the friends and the guys, but once I started to use more encouraging words when I talked to myself, I recognized there was no reason for me to continue communicating with those types of people, so I fell back from hanging out with them.

But wait, let me be honest: I did not always get it right when it came to the food for every single meal, and I still engaged with some guys I had no business talking to since I knew they did not have my best interests at heart. But I was wiser because I recognized that once a problem developed in my life, I did not wait like I did before for the wound to ooze, fester, turn green, and die to the point where I had to get an amputation. To maintain a normal life while losing all of this weight, I made an effort to plan out my workouts and meals, be flexible but firm when it came time to change up my routine once my work scheduled changed, get enough sleep, listen to my body's needs, establish a healthy relationship with food, spend time with my family, and speak with a therapist on a weekly to monthly basis to make sure I'm not being so hard on myself and embracing all the positive things occurring in my life.

I could have complained about all of the adjustments I had to make so that I could try to balance my two jobs and get in all of these workouts, but the truth is, the complaints would have fallen on deaf ears. Everyone I knew had 2 jobs, 2 kids, a spouse to take care of, they were going to school part-time, got a side hustle selling scented candles, and taking care of their dog named Felix who has heart worms. Everyone is busy, chile, trying to maneuver through this thing called life, and yet you still hear of people who lost weight on their own despite their circumstances. I was determined once and for all to master this journey so I could've had 3 jobs, a paper route, and 6.2 dogs to take care of and I still would have lost the weight. Without a doubt.

Any first sign of trouble that I knew would impact my routine, would be enough for me to eliminate it out of my life. You gotta remember, it took me years to craft this personal Iyanla Vanzant 'Fix Your Life' type of routine for myself. I came up with the perfect recipe to get out of my own way so that I could live life. And you think I was gonna let some man, a jealous coworker, or an associate sabotage my work? You were dropped like Latavia and LeToya from Destiny's Child with the quickness if you played those games with me. Nope, not this time. My mind was made up; I was fixated on being an active participant in my life, so I was willing to move at a moment's notice to correct any imbalances that deviated from such so I can stay firmly planted in the zone.

CHAPTER 9

POST-WEIGHT LOSS FITNESS ROUTINE

Mental Acceptance

Since I made the effort to incorporate my busier work schedule right into my healthy lifestyle, I continued to see results. When I wore pants, my legs now had room as I moved about (such a great feeling). When I walked up stairs, my stomach did not jiggle anymore. And most of all, I liked that when I climbed up a flight of stairs, I did not feel like I was going to pass out on that 9th step. Although I was winning at balancing my life, my weight loss started to slow down about a year into working the second job. On the weekdays that I worked at Bed Bath and Beyond, I was working from 7am to 10pm and getting home at 11pm. The 16 hour days were taking a toll on me, big time. I knew I was not getting in enough water, too, because you could not have drinks on the floor while servicing customers. Some nights I would have difficulty getting to sleep because I was going to sleep so late and still waking up early to go into my main job. I was still making my food and killing my workouts, but I was getting less creative with my workouts and was not challenging myself as much because I was exhausted.

Over the course of the next 2 to 3 years, I only lost about 10 more pounds. Within that time period, I quit Bed, Bath, and Beyond after working there for two years; it was time for me to go, chile. My weight loss now totaled 85 pounds, and after that I reached a plateau. I never thought I could lose even 15 pounds, so to lose 85 pounds was a huge accomplishment. Even though people, family, and friends were congratulating me and pointed out on a weekly basis that I lost weight, I was not entirely comfortable with the attention. It took a few more years for my mind to catch up to the fact that I was a smaller person. I went from a size 18 to a size 8 and I was mentally trying to accept that my body had changed. I was used to not looking in the mirror (I used to bypass any mirror with a vengeance) and now I would stare in the mirror somedays like, "Is this really you, Tasha?" I did not go out and buy a whole new wardrobe of skinny clothes because I was cautiously giving myself permission to mentally embrace the results of my new lifestyle. Losing so much weight caused anxiety for me at times because I looked totally different from the big girl I was in 7th grade and in college, and I was not sure if people genuinely cared about me or just made an effort to comment on it. So many people would come up to me and say how awesome I looked because I lost weight, and I took them as complements, but I also

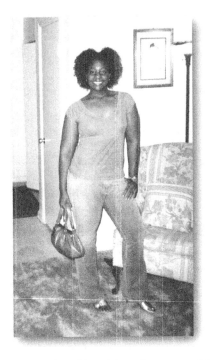

(Wayyyy more comfortable taking pictures at this stage
along the journey)

wondered why it took me losing weight for people to acknowledge that I was an awesome person. So now you want to acknowledge me because I lost some weight, but you did not even look my way 2 years ago? Hmph.

Once my weight loss became the talk of the circles I was involved in, it caused some people to question what I ate if we were together. They would look at me plating my food, what I ordered, and how I ate my food and this would cause my nerves to rattle. I'd get comments like "Is that all you're going to eat?" or "Where's the meat?" or "That's a lot of food you are eating" or "All you eat is rabbit food all day?" or "I could not do that, I'm a meat and potatoes type of guy," and maybe a few comments like "How are you eating that piece of cake and you're supposed to be Ms. healthy?" Meanwhile, I never tried to convert people to become a vegetarian or pescatarian, I'm just trying to get my little life together. So the comments were unneeded and sometimes taken to heart because I'm a sensitive person and I'm on this journey by myself. I learned that when you decide to go against the grain of the crowd, it causes frustration in other people because it makes them question what they are doing with their life. Some people became uncomfortable eating around me because they were eating the same food they were used to eating; they had their big plates of fatty protein and carbs on carbs on carbs, which caused a bit of self-reflection that could make some people feel a bit awkward. So I imagine the shame from my weight loss probably went both ways.

As for me, I could not enjoy myself as I used to because I felt like I was being put on display. All of my life I've been more of an introvert than extrovert. But this new-found weight loss caused me to want to "perform" in certain situations as opposed to "just live," and it was a bit draining. I mean, was I putting on a show in front of people about how I dressed and what I ate when I went to family functions and social outings? It made me question it all as I started to put pressure on myself because I felt this rising standard regarding how I was supposed to behave since I lost the weight. And as you know, I made a strong effort to not put pressure on myself once I started on this journey. So once I felt the pressure build up in my stomach from outside sources post-weight loss, it let anxiety creep back in to my life. I would not say I became anti-social, but I definitely was not signing up to be first at the club on Friday nights either. I just fell back and continued on my journey as quietly (but still efficiently) as possible.

In addition to people outside of me causing me to question myself, I had my own internal demons I had to deal with post-weight loss. I was scared as heck that I would wake up one day and my body would magically revert back to its original self. If you have usually been on the smaller side (even if you've gained 10 to 20 pounds in your life), then maybe you might have difficulty understanding where I am coming from. Ever since I was 2 years old, I've been characterized as obese in a society where being overweight is looked at as unkempt, lazy, and unattractive. When you live with those stereotypes day in and day out for most of the time that you have been living on this earth, you may start to believe some of those characteristics apply to you as well. Needless to say, I did not throw out any of my big girl clothes; I had to prepare myself in case I gained the weight back, chile.

I kept most of my bigger clothes for about 8 years post-weight loss. Eight years! Fear crept back into my life and it stuck around for a while. All I knew was struggle, what-ifs, and maybes, so I started to question whether I was even deserving of the weight loss. Looking back on those times, I wondered, "How could I even think that I would gain all of that weight back knowing how much work, sweat, planning and discipline I exerted to get to where I was?" I tell you, the mind is so fickle. I had no crazy boyfriend, parent, or friend say negative things to me like, "You know you're gonna gain the weight back" or "So you think you are better than me because you lost weight?" Nope, I had no downright negative people in my corner. All the Debby Downer what-ifs just came from me. In one instance, the mind can help you believe in yourself to start running on a regular basis and then 5 minutes later it can make you feel defeated until next January. Who knew that weight loss came with a host of mental emotions?

Nevertheless, I am glad I did not let my emotions overcome my actions to be an active participant in my life. Despite fear of the unknown and the pressure I was feeling from outside, like clockwork I still packed my sports bra, sneakers, leggings and 2 t-shirts to take with me to work out right after work. I was too far ahead to look back and revert. The thought to give up on myself occurred weekly in my brain as I was driving to the gym with the option to make a left and go home or to stop in the store after my workout to get a package of peanut butter Oreo cookies because I knew I was still in fat-burning mode and I could basically burn off half of those calories from the Oreos. The goal, however, was not to maintain, it was to overcome… I decided not to jump off the wagon because my routine had been set and I was crushing all of my opponents (the old me). I laid down the strongest foundation ever for success. My self-talk game was stronger than the random comments I received from people or the questionable thoughts I had for myself about my weight loss. I remembered how I felt being overweight and stifled for air just to exist. The current feelings I had were no comparison to what I went through in my past; this was lightweight and I needed to treat it as such. Plus, I was able to reap the benefits of my success by looking in the mirror every day. Yeah, I ain't go nowhere. Another killer leg workout followed by salmon, asparagus, and sweet potato coming right up for dinner, Tasha.

I BECAME A RUNNER

After losing all of this weight I see why so many people gain their weight back. It is not necessarily because they picked back up unhealthy eating habits and stopped working out. Well, that is part of it, but mostly it is because they were not mentally ready to accept what comes after you lose the weight. After losing the weight I was happy, anxious, scared, and nervous sometimes all in one day. Luckily, I'm a hard worker because that is exactly what is needed to maintain 85lbs of weight loss…a lot of hard work! I stuck to the plan I created, but I felt the need to add something new to the mix to help keep this weight off for life, so that is when I decided to add running to my fitness routine. Now let me tell you, I am the last person you would think of to start running. I did not like to run in gym class, I did not like to run to the car when it started raining, I did not like to play tag with kids in elementary school and I did not like running away from kids when they would tease me in elementary school. I got out of breath really quickly and I was not fast, so I tried to avoid running at all costs. When it came time to complete the physical education test in school, I would pass the running portion by the skin of my teeth. During high school, I played basketball and soccer but since there were so many other people on the court and field with me, you could not tell I was slow as molasses and about to pass out. I've always sucked at running, so it was surprising to me that I was even considering it.

I was content with lifting weights on a regular basis and hopping on my beloved elliptical to work up a good sweat. Additionally, I started to read articles talking about the benefits of running, in regard to weight loss that I decided to try it out and see if it brought any additional changes to my body. I mean, the worst that would happen is I'd stop it and continue on with the routine I'd already created for myself if I did not like it. The last time I ran was when I played basketball and soccer in high school, so here I am 10 years later attempting to run again.

When I first started running, I was not even running or jogging, I would trot around the track at Norview High School. I knew one lap around the entire track was a 1/4th of a mile and I could not even run that without stopping. So I would practice jogging from the start of a straightaway to the end of a straightaway without stopping, and then I'd walk the rest of the way around until I got back to that same straightaway. Once I realized I did not die from jogging those 100 meters, I added additional meters weekly until I was finally able to run 1 mile without stopping. Some weeks it would be harder for me to move from 1 and 1/4th miles to 1 and 1/2 miles, but I did not let it stop me from running altogether. I just took my time and ran my regular distance and pace, and then when my legs felt loose enough, I would continue my stride for a little longer to see if I would make it to the next 1/4 th or 1/2 mile. 9 times out of 10, I was able to make it to that next milestone, I just needed to attempt it. Running a mile without stopping was a totally amazing feeling. I shocked myself with this achievement as well because I thought you had to be a size 2 to run long distances.

When I started running, I was not on social media at the time so I was not able to connect with other black female runners or see runners with different body types hitting the pavement. I was just riding this high by myself until I got tired of it. The thing is, I never got tired of running. I kept running as a part of my weekly routine. I loved the high I felt after running 2, 3, or 4 miles. I loved the sweat I worked up while hitting the pavement. The sweat I worked up while using the elliptical was major, but the cardiovascular response my body received from running 3 miles was very different from the elliptical. And although the running was harder on the body than the elliptical, I felt that my body was challenged more from running. And if I was challenged more, I knew it would help me lose more weight. Once I got off the elliptical, I could move right on to my next workout or jump in the car to head home. After a run, I would have to collect myself before preceding to my next activity. I knew my body's performance and athleticism was increasing due to the weekly running, and I was *here* for it. Since there is no stopping point on how many miles you can run, I would test myself to see how many miles I could go without stopping. As you know, I was a sucker for a challenge and a new goal to add to my routine, so I got a thrill out of testing my body's capabilities. I did not start to weigh myself more often once I started running or try to find a running partner. I just decided to add it to my weekly fitness routine and leave the success up to how consistent I was with the running. Running became "my thing."

The enjoyment I got out of pushing my body to the limits was taken a step further when I started signing up to run in races. Soon enough, I was running in plenty of 5k (3 miles) and 8k (5 miles) races taking place weekly in Hampton Roads. My greatest feat came in 2009 when I signed up to run in the Rock and Roll Half Marathon. At this point, I was up to running 6, 7, and 8 miles, but nowhere near the 13 miles needed to complete the race. I still do not remember why in the ham sandwich I decided to run this race, why I paid money to run this long of a distance, or what was going through my head as I walked to the starting line of the race, but I decided to take my chances and give it all I had. I did not get a chance to run 13 miles prior to the race, but I've been in beast mode for years, stomping out every goal in my past so I was like, I can knock this out without the extra training! Yeah right, that definitely was not the smartest move I've made in my life and I paid for it...big time! The gun sounded, and we were off for 13.1 miles of hard labor (I mean running). There were thousands of people running right along with me so my adrenaline was pumping with excitement. I could not believe I was actually running in my first marathon so I was feeling myself...go Tash! You are the bomb, chile! I felt fine at mile 4, 5, and 6, running with a smile on my face at times and having a normal breathing rhythm. But then, once I completed mile 7, things started to go downhill. Once I reached mile 8 and knew I had 5 more miles to go, that is when I knew I was in way over my head; I knew I was not mentally and physically prepared to finish this race. Everything on my body felt like it was deteriorating and I started to gasp for breath as I took each stride. As I trotted along in the heat, I then began to think about all the bad decisions I made in my life and how the Lord must have been paying me back for them. I was not experiencing pain, but I felt like my body weighed 700 lbs. while trekking through the desert while carrying an 80lb backpack and wearing Timberland boots. By the 10th mile, I stopped. Now, I have never stopped running while training or participating in any of my other races. So even though I was tired, I still could not believe that I stopped. But I was more than tired, I was exhausted. In all of my years on earth, I had never felt more exhausted in my life than I felt at mile 10. Nevertheless, I had to pick up the pace so I could get out of this race, I was over it!

When I attempted to take off running to finish the race, that is when I knew I made the biggest mistake of my life (I should have never stopped running). As I put one foot in front of the other to run, I felt intense pain in my knees and ankles. Before the half marathon, I never experienced any type of pain while running, so my mind was trying to take in the fact that I was running a marathon, in pain, and there was nowhere in sight for me to sit down. I had to run those last 3 miles in severe pain and it was awful. 13 miles later, the race was over, and I knew first-hand what it felt like to almost visit Elizabeth, you know, Fred Sanford's wife in the TV show 'Sanford and Son?' Yeah, that was me on race day. I do not think I could ever thoroughly explain what I was feeling once I finished that race. My body was in a state of shock and it was trying to figure out what it needed do to heal itself, give me oxygen, and pump blood to my heart and legs without the use of pain medications, IVs, and surgery. I could not even walk; I had to take a golf cart back to my car. The rest of the day was a blur; I was overheated and in pain. I tried to take an ice bath to decrease the inflammation in my body, but I could not get comfortable enough to take the pain of sitting in ice for even a few minutes, so I just continued to ache for the next 36 hours.

Messages I took away from running the half-marathon:

1) You have to properly train for something of that magnitude so you do not die.
2) I am never doing that again in my life.
3) I am secure in what I have achieved thus far in life and have no desire to try another half marathon or a full marathon for that matter.
4) I'll stick to running my 5Ks and 8Ks – I am very content with that. Chile.

I continued to run as a part of my weekly fitness routine but not in races. I ran 3 miles about 3-4 times a week in addition to my strength training. The funny thing is

I got so caught up in running as a sport that I did not recognize what was happening to my body. The running helped me to drop a few extra pounds, but more importantly it helped me to reduce body fat. All of a sudden, I started to see definition in my shoulders, stomach, back and legs. It was as if the running helped to showcase all of the muscle I built up from lifting heavy weights these past few years. For me, the heart thumping, tired legs, achy calves, and sweaty mess I felt after running 3 miles was no comparison to the results my body was getting from running. I mean, for the first time in my life, I actually saw a muscle on my body; I did not even think that was virtually possible. I was amazed at the metamorphosis my body was going through; and the running helped to enhance that transformation, so I was hooked for life, chile.

So What Are You Going to Do With Your Life?

My body took such a turn with the running and muscle definition peeking through that people who did not even know me were coming up to me and asking if I was a trainer, did I run track, or if I worked out. When I started to get compliments from strangers, it gave me further confirmation that not only was I a smaller person, but I was a *fit*, smaller person. In the past, I just wanted to know what it felt like to be a smaller person. However, once I achieved this certain level of weight loss success, I realized that I started to desire a body that was strong as opposed to just small, and I started to encourage other women to add strength training to their fitness routines as well. Around this time period, I also started to re-evaluate my career and what in the ham sandwich I was going to do with my life. I was still working for the state at the disability office, just moseying on down the lane, but not really happy with what I was doing. My job enabled me to buy a car, a house, and pay my bills on time, but I did not feel like I was utilizing my talents in the right way. My job at disability was stable in terms of job security, demanding in terms of work, yet unfulfilling in terms of personal satisfaction. I toyed around with idea of moving out of the area, maybe to New York for a federal job or to Charlotte, NC, for a new job altogether, but when those moves did not occur, I knew that what I really needed was to satisfy this itch I'd been having concerning the start of my own business. There were basically three things that I wanted to achieve: I wanted to help people lead a better life, feel happy about where I went to work every day, and get back to starting this business that I dreamed about since I was in middle school.

One day when I was at work, I took out a sticky note and wrote down all the things that made me happy to see if I could create a living for myself while doing them. When I finished, I only had 3 things on the list (and in this exact order):

1) Sleeping
2) Baking
3) Working Out

Now as far as I know, no one can make money by sleeping. I wish it were possible because I love a good nap, but I could not make a dime while sleeping. The second was baking. As you remember, I've loved baking ever since I was a child. As I started to take on my healthier lifestyle, I found ways to "healthify" my desserts while still keeping in the flavor. I thought about opening up a bakery and/or selling my goods online to keep my overhead costs low. I knew all of the initial healthy cookies, brownies, and cheesecakes I was going to sell in my store because I've been baking them for years. But I decided to drop the idea of the bakery because I just was not comfortable at that time in being around food (and food that I loved) all day long. The idea of having chocolate chips, butter, flour, and cookie dough on my hands for most of the day in order to make a living was too much for me to handle. I did not want to take a chance and revert back to my old ways of overeating since I would be around my favorite foods all day long. So yeah, I dropped that particular idea after about a week.

The last thing on my list was working out. I absolutely loved being in the gym; it was my second home at that point and I could not get enough of it. The gym turned out to be a safe haven for me. I felt comfortable there, I found my mental and physical strength within those walls, and I realized there was far more to life than just what I had experienced thus far. My love for the gym prompted me to find out what type of career I could build within the fitness industry. The first position I saw was a group fitness instructor. Fitness instructors mostly got paid hourly by working in a big gym. Most traditional gym instructors taught class, on average about 2 - 3 times a day and about 2-3 times a week. When I watched fitness workouts on TV or when I popped in my workout videos to workout at home, the instructors were so vibrant, always had on a cute workout outfit, and were balls of energy for 60 minutes straight. I figured I could be that person to keep my participants up, moving, and engaged in their workouts, so I considered being a fitness instructor.

Upon doing my research, the fitness instructor gig was not gonna work for me for several reasons. Since instructors were most likely to get paid by the hour (as opposed to salaried), I knew that was not gonna cut it. When you carry the one and add the two, the money I made from being a fitness instructor was not going to be enough for me to make a living. I also did not feel that traditional fitness classes, often times, were as successful at physically transforming someone's life. Even on the front end, there is less commitment involved from the participant because they could attend class whenever the spirit hits them. More time, effort, and a strong relationship needed to be forged with the client and instructor in order for them to be successful at reaching and maintaining their weight loss goals, and that was not gonna happen in your traditional fitness classes. Lastly, I was not comfortable with working for someone. When I said I wanted to work for myself, that is exactly what I meant. I did not want to work full time at "Fitness-To-Go" and then work for myself part-time in the evening or on the weekends after I got off work – nah, that was not a part of the plan. I did not want to sell someone else's fitness nutritional guides or workout guides because I knew I could not 100% back their product since I did not have a hand in how it was developed. When so many people kept coming up to me to ask me how I lost weight and I recognized I could talk with them forever about fitness and weight loss, I knew I had something unique and powerful to share that came from *my* journey, not the journey of someone else. I was not looking for a side-hustle, I was looking for my own brand. My income had to come solely from my own mouth, hands, and effort, and it had to be all-encompassing of what people need to lose weight. So the fitness instructor position was off the table as well.

I then came across the occupation of a personal trainer. I did not really understand the concept of a personal trainer until I did a bit of research about what they provide to clients. Once I read up on how personal trainers "have the unique opportunity to adapt and individualize exercise workouts according to your clients' distinctive backgrounds and goals…in a safe and effective manner…," I knew this was what I wanted to provide.[10] I loved that there was a consistent, on-going relationship that needed to be established between the client and trainer. As someone who lost weight and struggled every step of the way, it was important to have an expert (not just a fitness enthusiast or a friend) who could guide you through all the highs and lows that come with attempting to lose weight. I loved that I could curtail my workouts to the person's current training level instead of giving a one-size fits all workout to everyone that wanted to work out with me. Since this was going to be my own business, I liked that I could charge clients what I felt was reasonable, not what the big gym decided for me to charge. So the personal trainer move was definitely on the short list.

Once I decided that I wanted to get into the fitness industry, I started reading everything about fitness, including articles on the health status of men and women in the United States. I found it particularly alarming that African American women are at a 50% higher rate of developing heart disease than any other race. According to the American Heart Association, African American women 20 years and older have a 50% chance of

---

10 Copyright © 2003 American Council On Exercise. All Rights Reserved. Reprinted by Permission.

developing heart disease. Black women are also dispro-
portionately affected by diabetes and stroke compared to
Hispanic women and white women. 1 in 4 black women
over 55 years of age has diabetes. The comforting news
I found in reading all of these statistics was that 80% of
the risk factors associated with these medical conditions
(i.e. obesity, high blood pressure, sedentary lifestyle, high
cholesterol) can be controlled by changing your lifestyle...
cue my company's appearance on to the scene![11] I'd been
searching for my "WHY" as to what role I wanted to play
in society and I found it. I was over the moon excited
that I found a career that I was excited about starting
and making my own while playing a profound role in
shaping the lives of African American women to lead
healthier lives. If I was able to reach my goals, there was
nothing keeping other African American women around
me from changing their life as well. And I knew that my
story about how I suffered with 2 of the risk factors for
over 20 years and overcame them through changing my
lifestyle would resonate well with clients because I am an
African American woman as well. It was then that I realized that I discovered what role I wanted to play in shaping the lives of my community while establishing myself
as a business owner.

---

11 U.S. Department of Health and Human Services, National Institute
of Health. The Heart Truth for Women. July 2009. http://www.nhlbi.
nih.gov/health/educational/hearttruth/downloads/pdf/factsheet-ac-
tionplan-aa.pdf

Heart disease, stroke, and diabetes affect all people in this country, but everywhere I turned, the numbers suggested that African American women are suffering much more from these conditions than anyone else, and I had to do something about it. My business was not going to be set up to only cater to African American women, but when alarming statistics hit you so hard about women of color who are suffering from such serious health conditions (some of which can be controlled), I knew that me being an African American woman who is knowledgeable in this health and fitness field could draw people in to change their lives. I saw first-hand from my own family members who were on several medications for their "pressure" and "sugar." I also had friends who spoke of the same common medical trends occurring in their own family. So this health issue was not just a trend or something that happened to other black women – these medical conditions were killing and affecting the well-being of my family and the family members of friends at a younger age than they should. African American women are the cornerstone of the African American community and if they are not well, then the community will also suffer. So that was that, I was going to be a personal trainer.

The second piece of this discovery was that I wanted to open my own business as a personal trainer. Now that I knew I wanted to be a personal trainer and that I wanted to make a living solely from doing it, I had to "businessfy" it (I know that's not a word). To me, that meant that I was not going to work for a gym. Initially, I did not even want to work part-time at a gym to gain some training because I did not feel they were really connected to helping people transform their bodies. I always felt their focus was on sales and getting as many people through the door as possible, regardless of whether they reached their goals or not. So I wanted to start off by creating my own business in order to open my own fitness studio in which to conduct my personal training. It sure would have been easier to work for a gym and then transition into opening my own studio. The gym would have laid the foundation about how I would conduct training, sales, advertising, scheduling, policies, pricing, insurance, legal affairs, etc. I was tired of working for The Man; I wanted to create my own rules, my own training style, my own policies, my own price structure, my own marketing scheme, my own business structure, and my own gym space. From now on, it had to be Tasha's way or no way.

The 85 pounds I lost on my own gave me the strength and confidence to step out and open a business (again on my own) that probably would not have come to fruition any other way. So instead of working for a gym, I immediately started to search the area for fitness studios and trainers that would let me shadow them while they trained their clients. Simultaneously, I looked around to see if someone would let me sublease space out of their studio so I could start to train clients. I searched around, and got a whole bunch of "sorry, I can't help you" responses until a guy named Kirk Allen from Genesis Fitness Studio allowed me to start training clients at his studio.

I continued to work for the state in Disability Services, but now I was working part-time as a personal trainer. I knew it was probably going to be hard opening my own business – and the truth is that it was harder than I ever thought. Some people might think being a personal trainer is easy because all you are doing is telling people what exercises to do. WRONG!

And I had the nerve to want to be a personal trainer and a business owner at the same time. Being the technician and the manager are two totally different things that each require time, effort, money, research, and skills to be successful. I studied and got my certification as a personal trainer from the American Council on Exercise. I also read a lot of books on Entrepreneurship and plenty of those "How to Start a Business" books, but I never found that perfect combination of a book assisting people who were trying to start a business in the fitness industry. I'd say it's a bit easier now to find information on starting up a fitness-based business given the easier access to information via social media; nevertheless, there is still a gap in the market on how to maneuver through the fitness terrain with ease. Being a business owner for 9 years running, I could write an entire book on becoming a personal trainer business owner, so I'll save all of that information for another time. But the truth is that wanting to open a business and then actually opening a business (with the end goal of opening a brick and mortar studio) are completely different, and that is something you really will not know you are ready for until you do it.

I contacted all my friends and family and told them to reach out to their friends and family to let them know that I'm now a personal trainer. I can not remember who my first client was, so I will not lie and make one up, but I was thankful when those first 2 or 3 clients took a chance and signed up to train with me, and they were all referred by family or friends. Although I read books on personal training, fitness, health, and entrepreneurship, I more so learned how to be a personal trainer and business owner while on-the-job. One would think since I immersed myself even further into the fitness field that I should have lost a ton more weight. UMM, NO. My time-management skills were being put to the test with this new routine, chile. Learning how to keep up with my schedule, the schedule of others, make sure workouts were scaled to each individual's training ability, check in with clients, assist with nutritional guidance of each client, and handle all of the business affairs was plain crazy. How in the ham sandwich was I supposed to do all of this by myself, work full-time at my other job, AND lose weight?

My schedule was jam packed with working my first job, then providing the service of my business, which consists of training the clients and running the business at the same time. In between those times, I was studying how to be a better trainer and learning how to run my business the most efficient and effective way possible. I loved giving people challenging workouts and helping people realize their potential. Even to this day, whenever I get a new client, I get excited about the possibilities of them changing their lives for the better, so the personal training portion of the learning curve was a little easier for me to comprehend. The business side was a different beast all together. I was uncomfortable talking with people about money, for starters. I did not like it at all, but I quickly realized that I needed more money to run the business and pay my bills so that I did not end up homeless. Instead of letting my business fail in the first few months by charging people $10 a training session, I spent money monthly on sales training. I paid $250 a month for about 6-7 months to a company that would teach me, once a week, how to ask people for money for my training sessions. Imagine having to pay money to get trained on how to ask people for money? It might seem silly, but I knew what my weaknesses were and if I was going to do this permanently, I had to ask for assistance to obtain profit.

Within 2 years of starting my business as a personal trainer, I decided that it was time to venture out on my own and open a personal training studio. I was not financially ready to open up the studio, but it was one of those things that I had to do because there was never going to be a perfect time to do it (*Is there ever a perfect time to reach your goals?*). So I stepped out on faith and opened up my own personal training studio. Even once I got the personal training studio open and running, I was still working full-time for the State. So my schedule would go something like this: Monday through Friday, I would train one to two clients from 5am to 6:30am, work at my full-time job from 7:00am to 3:30pm, and head back to the studio from 4:00pm to 8:30pm. Saturday: Personal Training from 8am to 12pm. Sunday: "Rest." I kept this insane rotation going for about a year until I quit working for the State and worked full-time solely bringing in income only from my business, T2 Fitness, in 2011.

During these three years, my body was probably all types of confused: it was working overtime seven days straight! I rarely had down time because I was working long hours most days of the week. I lost about 5 pounds over the course of these years. Obviously, my workout routine changed, so I was working out some days early in the morning and some days late at night. I dropped down from working out 5 days a week to 3-4 days a week. I was hauling food all over the place because I was rarely home. I was not eating out because I was always working. When I was not working, I was sleeping because I was tired from working. But I was not mad at all because I had my business doing what I love and it sure beat sitting in front of a desk 8 hours day staring at a computer doing something you are not connected to at all.

After my second year in the studio, my physique started to change again. The year before, I started to incorporate seafood back into my diet and I reduced my carbohydrate consumption. The increase in seafood protein and reduction in carbs leaned out my body even more to the point that I was sporting a two-pack honey (not six-pack abs, but more like a two-pack abs). The abs were just icing on the cake. Even though I only lost 5 pounds, it looked like I'd lost even more than that because my body fat percentage considerably went down. I did not get on "The Journey" to get a two-pack, but you best believe I'll take it!

So now that I lost 90lbs and became a business owner, I had to figure out how I was going to maintain this figure. If I thought finally losing weight was hard, then I had not seen a thing. As I look back on "The Journey," what felt like such a hard thing to achieve pales in comparison to what lies ahead. Maintaining a profound amount of weight loss is the hardest thing I've ever done and will probably be the hardest thing I will do in my lifetime. In order to maintain my weight each year, I sort of have to reinvent myself to garner a new type of strength, focus, and commitment. Each year brings about new challenges, hurdles, highs, and lows, and how I deal with them ends up affecting how I feel and therefore how I look. I had to get stronger, continue to have self-love, accept, adapt, and find a new way to get "in the zone" each and every year – and that is rough. I understand why people gain the weight that they worked so hard to lose back. Life throws so many curveballs at us that if you're not looking in the right direction, you can fall right on your butt and have to start the process all over again.

The tests I started to face as a newly-formed business owner were rough, but they were not going to cause me to revert back to the size 18 I was 8 years ago. I'd come too far to succumb now; there was no way I was turning back. My response to these tribulations was to devise a new routine (the reinvention) to keep this plan going. I wanted to enable clients to have flexibility with what times we could schedule their workouts. Since my training schedule changed from week to week, I had to be flexible but still consistent with my personal workout times changing from week to week. My routine consisted of me working out 4 times a week for 60 minutes each time, and I increased the amount of high intensity exercises that I was doing. I had to permanently drop from 5 to 3-4 workouts, so I needed to make sure my remaining workouts were challenging enough to get my heart rate way up, my muscles fatigued, and my metabolism in-check. It did not matter if it was Sunday evening, Tuesday at 5am or Friday at 6pm – I was getting in those workouts (high priority). As for food, I kept my staple breakfast items at the studio: oatmeal, a water heater to heat up my green tea and oatmeal, yogurt and almond milk in the refrigerator along with protein powder and peanut butter. In the mornings, I would bring any additional breakfast items if needed, like hard boiled eggs, fruit, or veggie sausage.

Like most trainers, my training schedule consisted of a split shift. I trained clients in the morning (before they had to go to work or school) and in the evening (after work or school). My midday was free from training, so 9 times out of 10, I would eat lunch at home and it would be a salad, the same as I took to work when I worked for Disability Services. I usually got home after 8pm in the evening and I would eat whatever seafood I picked up from the grocery store for the week along with whatever veggies I had on hand. I'd have a cheat dessert once a week and keep it moving. I helped myself to make good food choices whether I ate in the house or out of the house. For example, if I was going to be somewhere longer than 2 hours, then I made sure to have healthy food around to eat while I was there: this could be at the studio, at my house, at the car dealership waiting for an oil change, or at a doctor's appointment. I planned my meals to a "T." If I was running errands and did not have any food on me, I knew what convenience store I would visit to pick up a healthy snack to hold me over until my next meal. I allowed myself no excuses for workouts or meals as it simply was not an option in my mind. My life functioned as a non-playing athlete. I ate to fuel my workouts, to fuel my brain, and to fuel my long hours. If the food did not work with my lifestyle, I would not eat it because it would leave me sluggish and too tired to keep up with the demands of my schedule. If junk food cravings entered my mind, I questioned whether I was really hungry or just being greedy; 9 times out of 10, I was just being greedy and I reminded myself my body has no use for junk. *My body was not junk, so why would I feed myself junk?* The self-talk and healthy habits I developed over these transitional years, conditioned me to always focus on what my body needed, not what my mind wanted (*The mind can play tricks on you, chile*).

As a trainer, I did not allow myself to give clients bootleg workouts because I was tired or did not feel like it. To this day, I've only called out from training one time for one client, and it was on a Thursday at 5am. The only reason I could not make it was because I had a terrible headache and I did not think I could physically make the drive to the studio. Other than that, I've never cancelled an appointment. I have to be "on" at all times, engaged, enthusiastic, and communicative with my clients to keep them committed to reaching their goals. I also have to be "on" to help myself remember about the personal goals I've set out for myself, and I could not do that without practicing what I preach by working out and eating right as well.

Now, about 2 to 3 years into owning my own studio and being a personal trainer, group fitness instructor (conducting boot camps in the studio and offsite), developing online fitness training programs, hosting yearly community fitness events, and running my business (i.e. as a janitor, office manager, nutritional specialist, marketing coordinator, advertising specialist, bookkeeper, special projects coordinator, sales coordinator, retention specialist, health coach, social media intern, and counselor), the lifestyle started to take a toll on me. My life (and schedule) consisted of me solely owning and running a business and I would be working more hours than I ever thought existed in a week. It started to get very stressful. Delivering the service of training clients, running the business, and trying to take care of myself led me to revert back to old ways as well as develop new bad habits.

CHAPTER 10

THE START OF SOME HARD YEARS

POST WEIGHT LOSS, LIFE GOT REAL...

I BLAME ARLENE from my job at Disability Services. Ms. Arlene was one of the sweetest, toughest older ladies I've ever met. Arlene and I were the only two people in our office who had the same job, and she'd been in the position for quite some time so I often relied on her knowledge for support. One day, I went into her office puzzled about a case I was reviewing and she was eating some oatmeal raisin cookies. Being the cookie expert that I am, these cookies appeared to be big, moist, and heavenly looking. She asked me if I wanted one and I said, 'no thank you' with the quickness because it was not a "cheat meal" day. When she told me she got them from a grocery store, I definitely knew I was not going to have any and turned up my nose. I only ate cookies that came from specialty shops, so a grocery store cookie was out of the question. I could not waste my calories on a grocery store cookie, the nerve! But Ms. Arlene insisted about how delicious these cookies tasted and she asked me to just try a piece. I said alright because I wanted to stay in Arlene's good graces since she was helping me out in my position. I tasted the cookie and it was such a magical experience: those cookies were the bomb! I could not believe all this big cookie magic came from a grocery store. But here comes the kicker: the grocery store she got it from was less than 2 minutes from my house (Harris Teeter) ...and it stayed open 24 hours! *Kill me now.*

The next thing you know, I'm heading to Harris Teeter at 10:45pm on Wednesday to get these cookies. I'm not just eating 2 of these big cookies – no, they were the bomb and I would eat 5 to 6 of them at a time. This cookie binge went on for months. I was spending so much time in Harris Teeter looking at cookies that I also decided to try one of their personal sized cakes, which was just as delicious. One, two and sometimes even three times a week for about 7 to 8 months I was going back and forth to Harris Teeter like a big girl on a mission to save cookies and cakes around the world, only for them to go into my stomach before I hit the sheets. I was taking in all this sugar and I still had a two-pack, probably because I was so freaking busy and still killing my workouts. I felt like such a hypocrite because I was telling my clients to eat one thing and then I would go home and do another thing. I got so tired and started to feel pity on myself for coming home late at night after working 16 hours to save the world from obesity, heart disease, and diabetes only to have to cook my own food and take care of myself. So the cookies were the reward I deserved for getting up day after day to save the world.

My struggles with anxiety were starting to catch up with me again, too, as I started to have a difficult time relaxing from being on-the-go seven days a week. When you are a small business owner, you have no down time. There is ALWAYS something you should be doing to keep the business running, and it is even worse if you want your business to expand. For business owners who have a family, who work hard day in and day out to keep their business afloat while going home to their second job which consists of taking care of their family, there is at least a human element to it. You're getting back unconditional love in return from the family you designed. When running your own business as a single woman, often times you do not get love back. You pour and pour and pour and pour into others and people benefit from it, but they take those blessings and success and put it into their own lives, not the business owner's life. I'm not mad about that at all; that is why I went into business. But as a single woman running a business, you need love. I have love from my family all day long. My mother, hands down, is my biggest supporter in life in general. Single (or any business woman for that matter) business women are usually touted as some of the strongest women in the world, but that characteristic trait should not be mistaken for a lesser desire for love, check-ins, and support. In all that

I do, I would have loved an in-house support system to help me through the tough times (just like everyone else in this world). In my lifetime, I've functioned more-so out of a relationship with a man, as opposed to in a relationship and there are pros and cons to that.

The weight of carrying the business on my back also led me to a love affair with alcohol. Chile. I did not start drinking alcohol until about 31 years old. On my 30th birthday, I had my first grown folk's birthday party and drank Moscato, which was a big deal! I did not pick up an affection for drinking based on the party because Moscato was too sweet and I was not about all of those extra calories. I did not really like the taste of spirits like vodka and tequila. Brown liquor was just too hard for me and frankly tasted gawd awful. But then there was wine and champagne. Awwww, the good life! Several months after my night of Moscato drinking, a friend of mine put me on to drier wines which are less sweet and less calories than Moscato. It was then I started to appreciate the taste of dry wines and fell in love with Pinot Noir and Malbec. Who created wine? Wasn't it Jesus? Well, whoever created it is an absolute genius because it is just a wonderful creation. About 2 years later, I got into Brut Champagne, which is just heaven on Earth in a bottle.

So now I had three MAJOR vices going on in my world that I had access to 24 hours a day: the cookies, the birthday cake, and the wine. I did not know if these items were just really good or if I was just getting weaker based on all of the responsibilities that continually got added to my life because I'm a business owner. I feel it was probably a combination of the two that caused me to veer off track on different days and times after I lost the 90 pounds.

My days as a small business owner are consistently uneasy. It's a hard journey to maneuver through because even though the business continues to expand, I am still performing 80% of the tasks involved in running the business while conducting the training for my clients (… working on changing this now)! I am also a client myself and trying to maintain the healthiest lifestyle possible so I can keep my weight off. Despite all that I've learned and all that I teach my clients on a weekly basis, I still have issues with all three of these VICES. I do not feel that people should remove all junk food or temptations from their diet because it is unrealistic and we should be able to enjoy things we love. Also, I do not waste calories on things I do not truly love, no matter how good it looks. If it is not a fave of mine, it will get left on the tray, in the bag or thrown in the trash without hesitation. However, the vices that I do have cause me to overeat them when I choose to indulge. My brain does not understand the word moderation when it comes to champagne or home-made Oreo brownies (there is that addictive personality peaking through). I'm an all-or-nothing type of girl, and I cannot have just one glass of champagne or one brownie. No ma'am. I am going to want (and eat) 5 brownies and 4 glasses of champagne, and THEN I might be satisfied.

Evidence has suggested that sugar is highly addictive and that the body processes some forms of sugar in the same way the body responds to taking cocaine.[12] I've never tried cocaine, but I can tell you my body is sugar sensitive and becomes addicted to it once it hits my tongue. I feel that wine and champagne function as gateway drug once it enters my body. Once I drink a glass of wine or champagne, I instantly start to crave sugary and salty foods. The cravings come fast and hard, and next thing you know, I'm back at Harris Teeter trying to get my hands on some pita chips and hummus and/or cookies. I've heard people use a glass of wine as a form of relaxation to wind down after a long day and or as a compliment to their dinner. I've tried that, and yeah, it does not work for me. I would drink a glass of wine with my dinner and then eat a protein bar, an apple, and then bust out the house to get some tortilla chips and salsa and then look around like what just happened. Some weeks this might happen just once a week, but other

---

12 Sugar Addiction: Pushing the Drug-Sugar Analogy to the Limit. Current Opinion in Clinical Nutrition and Metabolic Care. https://www.ncbi.nlm.nih.gov/pubmed/?term=Sugar+addiction%3A+pushing+the+drug-sugar+analogy+to+the+limit
2013 Jul;16(4):434-9.

times it was happening 2 to 3 times a week and I was just in shambles. I would make my workouts even heavier during these times but it did not matter, the number of calories I was taking in heavily outweighed even the toughest of workouts.

I usually crave alcohol in the evening after one of my long 16-hour days. I usually have something I can eat for dinner at home, but my tiredness trumps the meal I have in my back pocket and I start to have a huge pity party for myself. I usually start to complain in my head and pile on all of the negative things going on (no matter if they are minute or not), which causes me to get pissed off. Okay, let me explain how a typical ride home on one of my long days plays out and ends on a sour note. My thought process would proceed through all of these statements in a matter of 2 minutes and end something like this:

- "I'm tired of doing all this by myself."
- "Working all of these hard hours, paying all this money in taxes and I still owe the government all this money in back taxes."
- "I trained 22 people today and I still didn't knock everything off my to-do list."
- "I can never keep up."
- "If I could have 2 more Tashas, I would be straight."
- "Everyone seems like they have a life and I'm just here "businessing" along."

- "For all I do, I should be further along in my career then I am now."
- "And after all of these years, why in the ham sandwich do I have to drive home and once I get there no one is there to build my life with."
- "I poured out everything I have to give today and I'm getting no love at home for this, ain't this a b%#$@."
- "Maybe I should get a dog."
- "Shoot, I ain't paying $642 for a random x-ray of the dog's left pinkie toe."
- "Man, let me just get some champagne and 5 cookies, write out my to-do list and go to bed for this 4:15am alarm for tomorrow."

Let me tell you, this same scenario has played out in my head about 125 times since I've opened up the studio and I just hate it. The day after my eating binge, I do not move as fast as I would like, I feel like lying in bed all day, definition in my stomach disappears, I'm not as productive as I usually am, I feel heavier, and I'm mad at myself for being hypocritical. Most importantly, I know the food does not solve a dag-on thing, yet I use it for short-term relief of my feelings. I blame Ms. Arlene for it all.

As a result of my stress and binges, my weight has fluctuated over the past 3 years. I did not consistently stay at 90lbs lost every single day of my life. My weight gain can fluctuate upwards anywhere from 5 to 15 lbs. In the past when I gained weight, I could bounce back in a week and the abs were tight. But since I turned 35, that bounce back phenomenon has vanished, honey. Despite the weight training, my metabolism has started to slow down, but the stress has not gone anywhere. Within the past year, post-binge can take me anywhere from 1 to 4 months to recover, so it's truly been a struggle for me.

So what am I currently doing now to combat these cravings, binges, and stressful bouts I go through weekly while being a single, recovering obese young woman turned fitness trainer and small business owner? *I don't give up.* The main reason why my business has remained intact during these stressful, crazy times is that every day I wake up and recognize that I have been given another chance to make better decisions than I did yesterday. I put in a substantial amount of effort the next day to change the trajectory of my actions. The next day I might win or the next day I might have another piece of cake, but the thing is that I try. I'm a friggin' fighter. I will try 427 different strategies to beat whatever I'm facing until I come up with a win. My mental game is a gift and a curse – it can get me down and only focus on the negative, but then it will look at the glass half full and find a way to make a way.

People always say "never say never." But I'm telling you right now, I will never give up on myself. NEVER. Just because the therapist diagnosed me with Major Depressive Disorder and I struggle with food, alcohol, loneliness, anxiousness, and stress every now and then while trying to take my business to the top is not indicative of what future success the Lord has in store for me or what I can mold my life into by even the end of this month. When I'm feeling off, in terms of my willpower to make healthy food choices, I take pity on myself for a day (or 3 days). But then I go into survival mode, take shelter, breathe, collect my thoughts and go a bit hardcore in my efforts to get back on track.

Some of things I do to get back "in the zone" consist of:

1) Intensify my workouts. My workouts are a bit harder in order to burn more calories and to knock some sense into myself. I'll increase the intensity of my cardio-based exercises and up the weight while doing legs or biceps.

2) I drink so much water that I'm floating to the bathroom every 38 minutes.

3) I cut off alcohol.

4) I put my debit/credit cards up so I am unable to make a run to the store while heading home from the studio.

5) I cut off social engagements if I'm not in a strong space to say no to alcohol.

6) I pray and ask God for peace, renewed strength and the discipline I need to carry out my day as honestly as possible.

7) Lastly, I do a ton of self-talk. I remind myself — while I am headed to grab something to eat or

while I'm actually eating — the reason why I am choosing to eat these healthy foods and its importance in me *living my best life.* I also talk to myself to get comfortable with the fact that I'm starting over.

I notice with my clients that starting over once they have gotten off track is one of the hardest things to do. I totally understand how it happens because it has happened to me so many times; you feel like a failure to a certain extent that you have to start all the way from the bottom. No one likes to feel like they are in last place. When those feelings start to creep in, I remind myself I'm not going to see results in a week and that is perfectly fine because that is not the main goal; the main goal is to reset your routine of fueling your body with food it needs to thrive and keep up with your demanding schedule. The aesthetic results will come because of the effort I'm used to putting into myself and the muscle memory that has come from lifting weights and running all these years. So I prep my food, knock out eating one healthy meal at a time and finish my workouts. Usually, if I can get through two entire days without my "cheats," then I know that I'm well on my way to getting back in the zone.

So you might be wondering, "What is your current health routine (sans the random dessert and wine binges) that has enabled you to keep these 90lbs off your frame for the past 15 years?" Welp, listen up because it goes a little something like this: I now work out 5 days a week and try to get in 60 minutes worth of strength training and cardiovascular exercise. It might seem like a lot, but it's only 5 hours out of the 168 hours in a given week and it is not a lot of time to devote to my health. My workouts consist of a combination of strength training (moderately heavy weight) and cardiovascular movements (boot camp drills, intervals on the elliptical, and running 1 to 3 miles whenever my body allows it). Since my body has been used to working out for the past 15 years, I know that the workouts I was doing 10 years ago will not elicit the same cardiorespiratory response today. So my workouts include a lot of combinations and a lot of weight. It does not matter if I'm out of town, under the weather, rehabbing an injury, or mentally drained from all of my responsibilities, Tasha will find a way to get in some type of physical activity. No excuses. I eat what I meal prep. I do not eat out on a regular basis at all – 90% of my meals in a month come from my house as opposed to a restaurant. My go-to snacks are almonds, apples, carrots and hummus, all berries (strawberries, blueberries, raspberries, blackberries, cherries), low carb protein bars, and protein shakes (vegan protein powder and unsweetened almond milk). I usually have one salty cheat food (pita chips, popcorn, or tortilla chips and guacamole) and one dessert cheat food (brownies, cookie, kettle corn popcorn, or birthday cake) each week and those portions are HUGE. Since I have difficulty managing the cravings, I only have alcohol on special occasions that are planned out in advance (i.e. My birthday, vacation out of town, holiday gathering, a close friend's birthday, or a wedding). After all of these years, those cravings still come on like a rampage and since I cannot control it, I cut it out.

Other than getting in some of my favorite cheats twice a week, I eat as clean as possible. My carbs mostly come from fruits, sweet potatoes, beans, and oatmeal. Bread is hardly in my diet – I only eat if I'm having brunch somewhere and I'm getting a crab cake benedict or avocado toast (those are my faves). Right now, I would be classified as a pescatarian (for all intents and pur-poses), so I eat seafood one to two times a day, eggs, and hardly any dairy. After being vegetarian for 8 years, I noticed that I gained more definition with seafood pro-tein as opposed to vegetable protein, so I added it back into my diet on a moderate basis. I aim to drink half my body weight in ounces. (So for example, if you weigh 250 pounds, you should aim to drink 125 ounces in water each day.) I faithfully drink hot green tea or a matcha green tea latte in the morning to wake me up for those 4am training times and to get my metabolism up from its slumber. I get 6 hours of sleep every night. Four or 5 hours of sleep gives me a headache and causes me to take in more calories during the day via snacking. I pay atten-tion to my hunger cues. I eat a lot considering I weight train 5 days a week and have long days – I'm always hun-gry. Therefore, I do not skip meals; I'd probably die if I did. If I know I'm going to be somewhere longer than 2 hours, there is ALWAYS a snack coming right along with me or I'll stop at a convenience store and pick up a snack with the quickness. I still do not indulge in alcohol on random weekends just because I made it to the weekend. My body does not look and feel its best after drinking and frankly it just does not work with me being a trainer, running a business, and all that that requires out of me every day. The alcohol slows me down (and keeps me bloated) too much to perform at my usual level. After following this routine for so long, it does not seem like work, that I'm being extra, or that I'm missing out on life. I've self-programed myself to live life this way (it is now an ingrained habit), it works, and I am content. Currently, I am a size 6, weigh around 155 pounds, very rarely get sick, and carry enough definition in my body to support my workouts and to feel and look comfortable in my clothes.

On any given day, there might be fluctuations in the portions of foods I eat (i.e. eating too much peanut butter), but this is my holy grail fitness routine that's been keeping my 90lb weight loss in check over these years. When I fall off in certain areas, I assess how well I'm doing with sticking to this plan and more times than not, I have veered off in some way from what I have written above. The quicker I get back to this routine, the more my weight, energy, and drive stays the same. Over the years, my fitness routine has changed based on my metabolism,

occupation, responsibilities, and convenience. I antici-
pate that this routine will continue to change throughout my life based on what is occurring at that time, and
I'm okay with that. Remember, I got into this knowing
that I was going on a journey, not a destination. I am
forever flexible while still committed to putting 100% of
my effort into making adaptations, changing my workout schedule, and finding different ways to incorporate
healthy food (and my cheat faves in moderation) into
my diet while maintaining a healthy lifestyle for the long
haul — that is how you stay on course and involved in
"The Journey."

C H A P T E R   1 1

❖ ❖ ❖

MEAL PREPPING

WHY AND HOW DO YOU MEAL PREP?

OMG THE FOOD is the hardest part! Ahhhhhhhhhh! I could work out every day until I'm blue in the face, but why do they have to make food taste so good? As you can tell from my past (and present) struggles, my relationship with food has had its share of ups and downs. Somedays, I feel like, "Man, I can never get it together, chile." My food relationship has gone from abusive, to obsessive, to comforting, to lonely, to structured, to healthy, and back to abusive, which does nothing but lead me away from internal peace. When I start to focus solely on the negative things going on in my life, my food choices tend to suffer. The truth is, while I've been on this journey, life has been occurring all around me and at one time or another, I've used food to deal with the stress. In each instance that I've used food to deal with my struggles, it has solved none of my financial issues, dating pitfalls, business decisions, heavy images of racism I've seen in the media every 4 months on Black people and minorities in our country, or family issues I have faced over the years. I've used food to overcome, process, and navigate through each of these issues at one time or another, and when I've finished inhaling that personal birthday cake from Harris Teeter, my issues are still there and the sadness creeps in. Other than curing hunger, food did not solve any one of my problems. Once I stopped obsessing over the fact that I made the decision to eat the food and accept that I'm not perfect (this could take an hour or up to several days), I thought about the severity of the issues I was facing. My thoughts turned from pity that I'm in the sunken place to holy hells bells, I'm sinking in this life boat and I need to start swimming ASAP! I started to assess whether or not I was obsessing, being extra, being moody for no freaking reason, I needed to talk to my mom or a friend about how I'm feeling, scheduled a meeting with my therapist, or just went ahead and put out the fire in that moment.

By entertaining a more encouraging conversation in my mind (which starts to turn down the volume on the negative thoughts) that focused on making a better decision when the next life-altering situation comes around, I was able to assess what self-made booby traps got in the way of properly fueling my body. More often than not, my answer to emotional overeating lied (and continues to lie) in my ability to confront what real issues I am facing…and plan my meals ahead, and that comes from meal prepping.

Why meal prepping? I know you've seen your favorite fitness enthusiasts on social media posting pictures of their meals prepped in containers for the week, wondering if it is really worth it to put in the effort. I'll tell you point blank, meal prepping is one of the ways I've been able to maintain my weight loss over all of these years. In Chapter 5, I mentioned how one of the 3 ways I stayed encouraged on this journey was planning out my fitness regimen, and a big piece of that had to do with meal prepping. The more time we spend at the last minute trying to decide what we are going to eat for that particular meal, the less of a chance you are going to make a healthy decision. I know my weakness was not failing to get in a killer work out, it was in making healthy food choices on a daily basis. So I made a conscious effort to spend time establishing a healthier relationship with food and devising a simple and cost-effective meal prepping strategy that I could maintain on a permanent basis. Meal prepping is annoying. Prepping can be interesting at times when I'm trying out new recipes, but often times than not, I would rather be doing something else with my time like taking a long Sunday afternoon nap. It's not one of those things that I'm looking to start loving anytime soon, but the truth is, if I waited to really like or love everything I did to lose these 100 pounds, I would not be where I am today. My feelings did not get me to where I am today; it's the effort, drive, and planning that helped me to establish a solid relationship with food.

Although I never feel like doing it, meal prepping has remained a part of my lifestyle because it works and it no longer requires substantial effort, it is a habit. I've been able to save time, money, and calories on a weekly basis for the past 15 years because I've made a conscious decision to meal prep. Meal prepping saves me time during the week because I do not have to mentally decide Tuesday evening when I'm driving home from the studio what I'm going to eat. I can re-heat my food, eat and move on to another task I need to complete before I hit the sheets instead of taking time to decide what to cook. Less time is spent during the week stopping at restaurants and grocery stores or preparing full meals when I take the time to meal prep on Sundays. As you know, my cravings tend to come in the evenings. If I'm one step ahead of the game and already know I have a meal at home, it increases the chances of me eating something beneficial to my body as opposed to picking up something unhealthy then feeling crappy once I wake up the next morning. In addition to saving time, I save money several ways by meal prepping. Generally speaking, we tend to spend less per meal when we cook (even if it's unhealthy food), as opposed to picking up lunch or dinner at a restaurant. You pay for the convenience of not having to prepare your meal once you decide to eat at a cafe or restaurant. Your lunch price includes the cost to make the food, the ingredients, and the containers that may or may not be used to store your food. When you pick up your items from the grocery store, we tend to buy our food in bulk so we get it at a cheaper rate. The price for food is less at grocery stores because you are the one that has to prepare the food instead of the chef (which is a time issue, but we will get to that in a minute). You also save money in the long run from meal prepping because you do not have to spend extra gas leaving your office during the day to pick up lunch or stopping in the evening to pick up food for dinner.

In terms of calories, meal prepping pushes you to make healthier choices during the week because you are deciding what to eat versus letting a restaurant decide what goes into your mouth. Maintaining supervision over your food choices also offers you more control over the portions of food you eat with your meals. For example, salads from restaurants over the years contain fewer vegetables than the salads I prepare at home. I'm more conscientious of the combinations of food that are included in my meals which is why they are healthier and better for me. I prep snacks as well because I'm a hardcore snacker. I love a good crunch, so I plan and prep what 2 snacks I'm going to eat so that I don't eat a whole bag of Skinny Pop popcorn at 4pm while driving back to the studio for evening training (I know who I am, chile). The more accessible healthy food is to me (i.e. in my refrigerator or cabinet), the easier it is for me to make a healthier choice for a given meal each day. I could be driving home and start thinking about what I'm going to eat, and once I start to think about my favorite cheats, a thought will pop into my head, "Remember, you still got the salmon and brussels sprouts in the fridge from Sunday." Next thing you know, I'm back in the game. Plus, I do not like to waste food! I'm not throwing away my precious little coins. If I buy it, I eat it.

There is not an official way to prep your food, but I suggest you plan it out as best as possible given the busyness of your schedule, the specific difficulties you face with eating healthy from day to day, and your budget. So how do I plan out my prepping from week to week? Okay, listen up. Here we go:

1) Decide on what day you will do your prep and put this day in your planner/calendar. I suggest prepping your food on Sunday or Monday as it is the start of the week. The later in the week you wait to prep, the increased chance you have at making a spontaneously unfavorable food choice and continuing that process for the remainder of the week.

2) Once Sunday rolls around, mentally decide what you want to eat for breakfast, lunch, dinner, and snacks. Breakfast items for me are still simple, require very little prep because I eat it while training at the studio, and usually bought in bulk so I do not have to buy those items every week (except for fruit and eggs). Right now, breakfast Monday-Friday consists of 4 different foods I interchange from day to day: 4 hard-boiled egg whites, 1/3rd of a cup of oatmeal, vegan protein shake, 1 piece of fruit (i.e. apple, grapefruit, berries, orange). I usually mix and match 2 of these items for breakfast all week; one item is usually a protein and the other item is a carbohydrate. (The protein keeps me satisfied until my next meal while the carbohydrate gives me energy to keep trucking on to perform the activities on my to-do list for the day.) On meal prep day, I boil 8-12 eggs and keep them

in the refrigerator for me to pick up as I'm running off in the morning to the studio. I buy a big canister of plain oats and keep it at the studio for me to eat when it's an oat day. If you are unsure of what you want to eat or are looking for a change up with breakfast, lunch, or dinner meals, Google some healthy menu items or check Pinterest and other social media outlets for new meal ideas. Do not be afraid of trying something new!

3) Head to the grocery store and pick up the ingredients you need to complete these meals. I ONLY purchase what I know I am going to eat for a week or for how many times I plan to eat a specific meal. I also only buy what my budget will allow.

4) Turn on music, cut, chop and get to cooking. I still usually stick to salads for lunch like I did when I initially started on "The Journey" because it is the best way for me to get in veggies at lunch and then I usually have lean protein and a ton of veggies for dinner. I also usually blast music from my speakers and get to dancing. Look, we gotta make this meal prepping thing as enjoyable as possible. So just embrace the time and effort it takes to get your meals done. Believe me, you will thank yourself once Wednesday evening rolls around!

5) Once you finish cooking, portion out meals into BPA-free single serve meal containers. Place snacks in sandwich bags and place additional grouped items such as extra veggies, chopped fruit, cooked

starches into large sized BPA free containers. For all of my smoothie lovers, if you are feeling like smoothies on some weeks, prep your smoothie mixes in freezer bags and store them in the freezer until you are ready to blend. I meal prep for up to 3 days at a time, but you can do it for the whole week if needed. If you are meal prepping for a whole week, I suggest you put your meals that will be eaten later in the week in the freezer, so they can retain their freshness. Then the day before you are ready to eat, take them out of the freezer and place them in the refrigerator before it is time to re-heat.

FIGURE OUT YOUR STAPLE FOODS AND WHAT NEEDS TO CHANGE FROM WEEK TO WEEK.

I need variety to stay consistent in this healthy food game (but if you want to keep your meals the same because it helps you stay consistent, then roll with it). Week to week, I rotate 3 different vegetables in my salads and a protein. As I'm writing this chapter, my lunch salad veggies for the week consist of broccoli, chickpeas, and red peppers. Once I get home from the grocery store, I chop up all of my lettuce and put in a big glass bowl. Next, I chop up my salad veggies and put them altogether in another glass container. So when it is time for lunch, I take out my salad bowl and take a handful of lettuce and veggies from my meal and place in the bowl. I top with my protein and I eat. That is it. I might also add that red onion, eggs, and avocado are staples in my fridge; they are used for omelets on the weekend, lunch in my salads, and side dishes for my dinner. Once any staple items run out, I'm heading right back to the grocery store to pick them up (and don't say you can't do this either. Last time I checked, a large number of people in this country live with a grocery store no more than 1-3 miles from their house or job and most of us have automobiles and/or feet, so don't try it!). The following week, my lunch salad veggies will change to keep the variety, texture, and crunch popping in my salads. Protein for my salads is also switched up from week to week and includes any of the following: crab cake, wild-caught salmon, smoked salmon, tuna from a can, wild-caught shrimp, veggie burger, or eggs & hummus. Remember, I don't buy all of these each week, I just buy enough for how much I am going to eat for that particular week.

As for dinner, I still cook 3 different veggie sides and 2 proteins at the beginning of the week (if it ain't broke then don't fix it) and place it into containers. Once the week is over, I swap out those veggies for different veggies for the next week. Spices and seasonings do not have to be purchased every week, but I buy my protein every week. Veggies for dinner are purchased either fresh or frozen (sans the ones that include a butter sauce) as they are both healthy. I always look to see what fresh veggies are on sale and in season (which means they are cheaper) since that also plays a role in what I'm going to cook for the week. Veggies are bought and portioned out based on how many days I plan to eat it. I usually can eat a meal/food up to 3 times; after that it's a wrap; so I never buy more of anything that will be eaten more than 3 days. I usually purchase two different seafood proteins a week that are wild caught and cost no more than $9.99/lb. As soon as I get home from the grocery store, I cut the fish into 3 portions, season, cook and put into containers. I don't cook all of my protein at one time since it is seafood. For instance, I'll cook enough salmon for 3 days worth of meals, and once Wednesday rolls around, I cook cod to finish out the rest of the week. Since I only spend up to $10 per pound, each protein per meal only costs me $3.33 or less a serving, which is way cheaper than if I went to a Ruby Tuesday's and spent $16.99+ tax on their Hickory Bourbon Salmon dinner (although their Bourbon salmon does taste good, chile).

If I want to try to create a new meal based off of something I found on social media, I check out the ingredients and recipe to see if I want to put the effort and money into making it. If you are new to the meal prep game, I do not suggest making anything too fancy, anything that requires 10+ different ingredients or ingredients that you know you cannot transfer to another meal. I also do not suggest cooking more than one new meal a week; all of these things can be overwhelming for you to follow through which could dissuade you from wanting to do this every week. To cut costs, try out your new meals on weeks you have more disposable income in case you are not fond of the meal to eat a second and third day. My goal with dinner is to establish staple meals, but 1-3 times out of the month step out of my comfort zone and try something new to increase the variety of meals I have up my sleeves. You have to establish some balance and comfort in the idea of meal prepping. Do not pile on the difficulty of your prep so it becomes overwhelming for you to perform from week to week, but put effort into trying something new. We gotta enjoy our food along the journey in order to remain permanently successful.

The weekends, like most people, can be complicated because my work/leisure schedule changes on Friday, Saturday, and Sunday. Nevertheless, I recognized that I needed some order when it comes to the weekend so I'm not pissed off at life about food decisions I made once I wake up Monday morning. I hated the fact of starting over on Monday, so I had to make an effort to do some prepping/planning for the weekend. Breakfast on the weekends is a little more elaborate, but is mostly made from unused items I purchased from meal prep on Sundays: omelets, frittatas, veggies, avocado, sweet potato hash, cooked apples, low carb breads/muffins, veggie sausage patties (only eaten once a week since it is a processed food), hummus, fruit, etc. Lunch is usually still a salad regardless if I'm eating at home or if I'm meeting up with a friend. Friday nights are eaten out but usually healthier foods: salmon, crab cake, 2 veggies. I often drink Kombucha during the weekend to starve off alcohol cravings. Kombucha is fermented tea that has been known to contain healthy bacteria such as probiotics and helps to support our immune system. Besides the health benefits of Kombucha, it is usually low in sugar and contains some carbonation so it helps to address the champagne cravings I get from week to week. Now on Sunday afternoons, a cheat meal is definitely consumed: 5 brownies, 2 big slices of birthday cake, chips, guacamole, champagne (if it's a special occasion), nachos... just whatever I'm feeling for that week. Weekends I usually allow myself one 32-ounce fountain Cherry Coke Zero (I know it's bad, but look, I love it so whatevs). Depending on how strong my food game has been the past week and where I meet up with people later on to socialize, I might eat before I head out. I do this for two reasons:

a) If I've been having difficulty that week hitting my food marks, I'm doubtful of making healthy decisions when I go out, so I'll eat beforehand. At this point in life, I cannot afford to worry about whatever someone else feels about what I decide to put in my stomach. So I eat beforehand and just go to chat it up with the girls. (s/n: a true friend or spouse won't take it personally if you are trying to get your life together).

b) If I think a veggie or protein is about to go bad in the fridge, I'll eat what I have on hand instead of at the restaurant so I'm not wasteful of my money.

I look at getting together with friends as more about the fellowship than about haphazardly taking in 1200 calories within a 2-hour time frame. My friends are not a part of "The Journey," it's just me. I'm the one that has to deal with my feelings once I leave them for the night, so I gotta take care of me first.

I also want to share a few random tips on what I've done to reap the weight loss benefits from prepping my meals the past few years.

1) The WHY? Consistency. I did not start meal prepping to lose a certain amount of weight. I started it to help me stay consistent with choosing healthier options and, as a result, the weight came off.

2) Do not incorporate every new, trendy food or diet just because its "healthy." Choose items you genuinely are interested in trying out and eating. I do not eat foods just because they are "healthy" or trendy; if the taste does not resonate with me, then I do not buy it (Lord knows I cannot stand turnip greens). I only try out one new meal a week. The less pressure I put on myself the better.

3) Buy glass, ceramic, or stainless-steel food containers; they're BPA free, which means they are made with less chemicals than regular plastic containers.

4) Buy a food scale and a new measuring cup to initially determine portions for carbs and protein (I eat as many non-starchy vegetables as I like).

Once I visually saw what 6 ounces of salmon looked like, I had a better idea about how I was portioning out my fish.

5) Don't be wasteful. Purchase what you know you can eat in a week unless you know some of the fruits and veggies can last longer than that. I always question clients who say, "My fruit and vegetables always goes bad before I eat it." My response is something along the lines of, "Well, if you ate what you purchased from day to day instead of deciding to eat out for lunch or dinner several times a week, nothing would go to waste." Buy what you know you are going to eat and do not waver once that food enters your shopping cart.

6) After you finish your prepared meal or snack, you should feel satisfied, not full. If you feel that you are truly still hungry once you finish your meal or snack, then I suggest you add more food to your meal on your next prep. Remember, being healthy does not always mean we eat less. Food is fuel, so each meal should keep hunger at bay until it is time for your next snack or meal.

7) Variety is important to me. Although I'm a creature of habit, I change up my veggies, carbs, and proteins from week to week. Peruse the produce section again and open your eyes to new possibilities. Most times, people have a restricted lens on

what they think tastes good, but you might not realize that your taste buds may have changed over the years if you are not open to trying something new. (S/n: ever since Rudy Huxtable from *The Cosby Show* declared brussel sprouts were nasty, you would not catch me eating them. But now 20 years later, I'm in LOVE with them!) If I had salmon last week, I'm not going to purchase it again the following week. If there is a wild caught piece of fish that is on sale and I'm not used to cooking it, I'll take out my phone and see if there are any recipes I'm willing to try out to take advantage of the sale.

8) Herbs, Season and Marinade (This is very important!). Along with the variety in my protein and veggies comes variety in how I flavor my food. I'm a foodie, so I like to try meals from various regions around the world. It was important for my meals to have some flavor to them in order to keep my international palette satisfied all these years. I took an interest in learning about the ingredients involved in preparing certain flavored dishes (via social media/YouTube) and applied that knowledge to my salmon, spaghetti squash, and quinoa. Whole Foods has a spice wall that contains a ton of different spices and seasonings that you can purchase by the ounce. I usually head there to try out new spices at a cheap rate

and decide which ones I want to add into my holy grail of seasonings. Once I season, I marinade. Since I do not like to add a ton of oil, butter, or cream to my meals (to keep my fat content to a reasonable level), I find that marinating my food really adds in the flavor to my meals. Also, since my meals are not eaten as soon as they are prepared, it gives the food time to really absorb the spices.

9) When all else fails, mentally plan out your meals. We all know that eating is the main thing we do several times a day, every single day of our lives. So stop being surprised when it comes time for you to eat, be mentally prepared! If for some reason, I do not meal prep for the week, you best believe I still mentally plan what I'm going to eat for each meal. All common sense does not get thrown out the window because I did not make it to the grocery store on Sunday. Not prepping out my meals is never an excuse for me to turn to Wendy's and order a fish sandwich and French fries. I know what I need to properly fuel my body. This is my lifestyle no matter what circumstances I may face from week to week, so I always attempt to make the best decision possible, prep or no prep.

CHAPTER 12

HOW I LOST THOSE LAST 10LBS?

WHAT DID I DO?

WHEN I INITIALLY started on my weight loss journey, I was 22 years old, very sedentary, questioning my WHY in life, and had youth on my side. Now, as I found myself yearning to lose these last 10 pounds once and for all, I needed to take into consideration where I was at present day. I'm a 37-year-old woman who is very physically active on a weekly basis with a metabolism that is dropping, stressed the hells bells out on more days than I would like, with way more responsibility thanks to me running a business and not enough time in the day. With this frame of reference in mind, I knew my strategy to losing these 10 pounds had to change from what I initially did to lose weight and what I was doing to maintain my weight loss. Since I knew I had to somewhat overhaul my current fitness lifestyle to reach this goal, I was not ready to fully commit to the process. In fact, in the past 12 months of my life, I went through a period of lows where I was so mad because the futile attempts I made to lose the weight were not successful. I could not drop weight like I did in the past, and as a result, I started to gain weight. I gained weight because I was upset that my body could not transform the way it did in the past, so I started to cheat more than just twice a week. Once again, I started to enjoy junk food (and hefty portions of it) 3 or 4 times out of the week (like that was helpful, SMH). In the end, I gained about 10-12 pounds over the past 12 months. *I let myself go...* So instead of needing to lose 10 pounds, I honestly had to push harder to lose 20lbs: the struggle has now risen to an all-time epic level.

Looking back, I know I self-sabotaged some of my efforts because I felt that since I have 48 things going on right now (which includes being a "healthier" person/ advocate), I should not have to work so hard to lose weight. Shoot, cut me some slack! Once I saw the weight was not coming off as I deemed it should, I decided to pile on the pity, chile. I still consistently worked out, but my eating was horrible. My clothes started to fit a bit too snug and felt uncomfortable. At the same time this was going on, I was still itching to reach this personal goal I've had for a long time and I knew deep down in my heart I could do it. I just was not mentally prepared to make it a reality, so I sat back ate my kettle corn popcorn and champagne and waited. I waited until I got totally uncomfortable. I was uncomfortable with starting over tomorrow; uncomfortable with my clothes getting tighter; uncomfortable that I was teaching my clients how to live a healthier lifestyle when my foundation was breaking at its core and I'm not following my own advice; uncomfortable that my routines and habits I built up over time were not being

followed like they did for the past 15 years; and uncomfortable that I was not comfortable in my skin. I still got
up at 4am to train clients, carried out all my responsibilities, put in my 16 hour days, smiled in people's faces,
danced whenever my song came on the radio (By now
can you tell I love to dance?), yet I was uncomfortable
with the direction I was letting myself get to.

After yo-yoing back and forth for the past 12 months, I
decided to face reality; I was in a semi-sunken place. I was
tired, drained, burnt-out, and over myself and this weight
gain, my schedule, and these reckless eating habits were
not solving a got dag-on thing. To close up the emotional
and physical wound that developed in the past 12 months
so I could drop this weight, I realized that I needed to get to
the root of the problem. I could not just say, "Okay Tasha,
you are going to eat healthier and drink more water."
Nope, that was not working this time around because later
that evening, around 8:42pm, I would still end up in Harris
Teeter's parking lot getting my birthday cake. Instead, I
needed to go underneath the surface to get to the root of
the problem. To lose 10 lbs at this stage in my life would
take a different kind of effort than it did 15 years ago and I
needed to be able to mentally embrace this train of thought.
My time is limited and my responsibilities require a lot out
of me that I cannot give to losing weight like I did in the
past. Plus, I am much smaller now than I was 15 years ago,
so that sense of urgency is not present. As I stated before, I
was emotionally drained and over continually feeling this

way from week to week. The exhaustion was preventing me from seeing clear enough to even think about a weight loss plan, so I started to assess ways to correct these feelings, not how to lose the weight. I did not sit down at the table and determine how I was going to remove the emotional baggage, I just started to think about it. I could be walking to my car, on the elliptical, soon as I'm getting out of bed, or while I'm in a group chat with friends. Whenever the spirit hit me, I started to think about ways to lessen my physical and mental workload.

STEP 1: GET AN ASSISTANT

The first solution I implemented to remove the emotional baggage from my mind was to have another trainer assist me with training clients. I was getting burnt out with keeping up with clients and running my business, so I decided to help myself out (I saved my little coins up so I could hire someone on a permanent basis) and got some help with training. While the trainer was at the studio, this freed up my time in the evenings to focus on other areas of the business that were causing me anxiety because they were not getting the attention it needed.

STEP 2: DECREASE PERSONAL TRAINING

Second, I decided to decrease my availability for 5am start times on Mondays and Fridays and cut off response times to clients after 9pm. This may not seem like a big thing, but it was HUGE to me. To this day, clients will still ask if I'm working 5am/6am on Monday and Friday or contact me after 9pm (now I put my phone on DO NOT DISTURB after 9pm). My phone chirps, tweets, or vibrates about 20 out of 24 hours a day, and it was getting to me. Sometimes I feel bad about the decreased response I give to clients, but the truth is that the "no" helps me to be stronger and a bit more focused for my clients and my own sanity. Also, my business does not consist of me operating on people in the emergency room, so they will be alright waiting for a response.

STEP 3: "ME" TIME AROUND THE WORLD

Third, I made sure that I book one exploratory international trip each year. I'm not talking about going to the Caribbean or an island (which is still a great trip), but rather to another country to learn about the culture of people living life differently than me. The international trip was important to me because I feel that my career always gets the focus, which can cause me to be very self-centered (primarily because I am responsible for a lot by myself), and I want to remain humble while learning from people that are outside my usual sources of influence. Also, planning an international trip I get through the daily business owner grind reminds me that I'm not just working to work.

STEP 4: SWEAT IT OUT

Fourth, I added in hot yoga to my weekly routine. Hot Yoga refers to yoga exercises (or postures) that are performed in a room up to 104 degrees Fahrenheit. The benefits for me to performing hot yoga are to lessen tension around my back (which gives me pain from time to time) and also provides me that post-yoga excess drainage to help relieve stress and toxins from my body. Although performing hot yoga has forced me to wear hats way more than I would like to because my natural hair is drenched after each session, I feel more relaxed and able to sleep better on my hot yoga days. More sleep for me means less time worrying about things out of my reach, establishing a better sleep pattern and waking up with a clearer focus to take on the tasks of my day.

STEP 5: ASSESS FRIENDSHIPS

Fifth, my mental anguish led me to assess my friendships with women and men. Okay, so here are a couple of points on how I interact with friends. I feel like since I've always been so much in my head, I've never been one to entertain drama filled people; I'm allergic to drama. It's rare that I have drama with girlfriends. If you are "extra," it's a 100% chance we are not friends because that is just too much for my soul (I do not even watch reality TV shows because the negative dialogue and behavior is just too much for my spirit, and I absolutely hate how it makes African American women look to the world). Because I care so much for my friends, it comes natural for me to check in with them regularly to make sure they are on the up and up. However, during this time of mental refocus, the main thing I've done to get to a moment of clarity is to not put pressure on myself to check in with everyone all the time. It is my hope that my friends remember my character and how we have carried our friendship over the years to know that I love them no matter how much we talk so I could get my little self back together. And again, I know my girlfriends are busy themselves, so there's a 92% chance they're not worrying about me either; it is usually just all in my head.

Luckily, I've always had good girlfriends who recognizes me as someone who has their back and cares about their best interest, so quarrels with girlfriends are a rare occurrence. Now leading up to the point, if you caused me to question your real intentions and started to take me for granted then I'll either say how I feel and peace out, or I'll just start to back away from you like Homer Simpson did into those bushes. If I notice I'm the one always contacting you, I made an effort to scale back while I've been in transition. During this time period, I chose whichever strategy required the least effort out of me to take on while enabling me to maintain friendships with friends that were equally beneficial to the growth process for both of us.

Guys are another beast all of their own that required an actual assessment. SMH. I will give guys several chances (because I know they are from another planet and do not operate in the same fashion as women) to correct their efforts, and ALL of them who I've been involved with will agree that they needed to put in more effort. To be honest, I just think most of the single men (whether we are just friends or attempting to date) I meet are just coasting. Most men around my age, give or take 10-12 years, are just riding the wagon until the wheels fall off and I see why. One, there are plenty of women available to them in these streets; therefore, effort has gone by the wayside because its unnecessary. Two, the misinterpretation in society of the independent woman has caused some men to think some women do not desire a true partner in life. If you are taking care of yourself (as I should be because I'm an adult with bills and ambition), somehow this has become translated by society that I am intimidating and/ or do not desire the love, companionship, assistance, and bond that could be obtained from a man. Three, just like women, men have obtained baggage over the years from dealing with women (we can be bat crazy), which causes their trust with women to somehow dissolve for the next 42 years. And, from what I hear from men, they get tired of 'adulting' as well, so they just ride the wave, chile.

So what does all of this mean in terms of my interactions with a lot of men? It means whenever the wind hits them, they will fly in that direction until another breeze comes which forces them to shift gears in another direction. This toss and turn guide seems to work well for most of the guys I meet, and that is cool if it works for them. I, on the other hand, cannot be swayed by wind, hail, or hurricanes (no matter what has happened in my past), so it presents a bit of a conundrum for my brain on how to interact with these types of guys. I know who I am and that I want someone of added value and consistently involved in my life (whether we are friends or soulmates). So if I noticed a pattern that you are not at the stage of providing consistency and effort (which does not have to match mine but is persistent) to me when I know I'm giving that to you (in addition to all I have going on), then they got dropped during this stage as well. I'm still cool with these guys, but nah, you are not qualified to even hover around my circle. Look, it is real out here in these streets.

PUT THE FORK DOWN AND ASSESS EVERYTHING

See, before I developed a strategy on what I needed to restructure in terms of diet and exercise, I went through an assessment of everything else I was putting effort into in my life to determine whether I needed to remove it, decrease it, or switch it out with something more beneficial to my progress. More often times than not, I realized I had to drop and switch. I dropped bad habits and bad people. I dropped the number of hours I devoted to actual training. I dropped my training times so I could improve the efficiency and upward mobility of my business. Basically, I was carrying too much unnecessary stuff. Since I dropped my hours, I had to shell out more money (Who does that? Who even wants to give up money?), so I could be more restful to handle various tasks that come my way. I also dropped the amount I was running (which was saddening) and switched to hot yoga to lessen lower back tension and give me a more restful sleep. I dropped the amount of pressure I was putting on myself to make sure I was being a nice person to girlfriends and guys and switched to thinking about myself first; shoot, that is what everyone else does. By me dropping and switching my thought patterns and habits, it allowed me to mentally clear the way for more change in my life. I was still busy as crap and these adjustments did not make it easier for me to lose the 10lbs. However, the changes brought about the mental cleansing I needed for clarity and a restructuring within my spirit to transform my body once again. I was now mentally equipped to lose weight.

Now, back to the harsh reality of it all: it was harder to lose weight now than it was previously. Ughhhhh. Foods I could "cheat" with and still lose weight in the past were not working this time around and that pissed me off. I'm 15 years older than I was when I started on my journey, so my body has changed. How do I know? Because even though I've been working towards losing weight and saw some change, I do not have the muscle definition I had when I was 30 years old. The internal makeup of my body has changed, in other words, and I needed to get over that quickly. My body is slower to respond to whatever stress load I put on it and I needed to put in more consistent effort than I had in the past 8 years. Also, no matter the routine and structure I come up with to lose these 10lbs, this weight loss is going to be an inconvenient goal for me to achieve right now. I legit have no extra time on my hands to lose weight. Even so, it must be done, and in order to lose weight this time around, I realized I needed to have patience and discipline.

PATIENCE

The words "Patience" and "Discipline" are the only 2 words I have up in my studio and have been my mantra for the past 2 years. Patience and discipline are the quint-essential keys to reaching any type of goal in life and this is also true when it comes to weight loss. I realized that I was not going to be able to drop weight quickly just by running, lifting weights, and eating healthy anymore because the truth is that I'm busy. From 4am until 8pm on most days of the week, my mental and physical work-load was being utilized to keep my business running, progressing, and expanding; therefore, I have to share my energy between running a business and implement-ing a plan to drop these last 10 lbs. Since energy is not infinite and it must be shared, it might take me longer to lose the weight and I started to be okay with that. I recognized that my patience was going to be tested all throughout this journey because in order for me to see change, I was going to have to work harder than I normally do, and that is some hard stuff. I had to work even harder because my body is used to working out, used to eating healthy, and used to working 16 hour days. My body has gotten into this cushiony health-kick groove, so stepping it up even more was going to require patience on my part to adjust to a new weight loss strategy.

DISCIPLINE

Maintaining discipline was going to be even harder than increasing my patience. According to Webster, Discipline can loosely be defined as *the suppression of one's desires, by enacting rules and utilizing self-restraint, in order to gain control.* I know what it takes to lose weight – I've seen it in my own body over the past 15 years and have witnessed it occur time and time again with my clients. I know that in order to lose these 10 lbs, I will have to maintain a high level of order and willpower to find success. And the truth is, my new "normal" consists of me working hard, and having to work even harder by myself while running the business on my own was a lot to take in (hence the reason why I was like "F it" last year, ate my cookies and took several seats). I was over it because I was uncomfortable physically and mentally with where I was. In order to win at this game, you have got to be uncomfortable with where you stand. Right now, I was itching in my seat, biting my bottom lip, legs fidgeting, eyes narrowing in and envisioning myself dropping these pounds every extra second of my day. I was totally uncomfortable and yearning for the structure and order needed to drop this weight and feel like myself again. I stopped feeling sorry for myself and proceeded to mentally put myself on the highest pedestal known to man. I deserved more self-love and life. 12 months later, I was ready to work.

It took me 2 months to do what I could have done 12 months ago, but I'm not mad, because I lost those 10 lbs, honey! I'm just glad that I did not give up on myself this time around and got it done. Since I was mentally ready to accept the patience and discipline that was needed to lose the weight, what did I actually change in my day-to-day routine to lose the weight? Here are the five strategies I used to maneuver through every hour in the 60 days it took for me to drop those final 10 pounds.

#1 WORKOUT MAKEOVER: BREAK IT UP

A total of 60 minutes of intense activity 5 days a week, completed over the course of a day, as opposed to at one time. My workouts usually last for 60 to 75 minutes; however, I was realized that I was not finishing all of the exercises in my routine because another client would come in and I would need to stop and get them started on their workout. Thereafter, I would just forego the rest of my workout and move on to other things I needed to get done for the day. Now what I did was break my workout up over the course of a day. For example, I would get in 25 minutes on the elliptical at 6am, 30 minutes of strength training at 8:30am, and then ran one mile in the evening 10 minutes before my 7:30pm bootcamp class started. Since I allowed myself to break up my workouts, I found that on some days I got even more exercise without effort. With the extra activity, some days I was also getting in 2-3 showers a day, and I wore my hair in twists throughout this time. By becoming a little less structured with my workout times (and more flexible with my sweaty times), I was actually able to become more physically active throughout the course of the day which increased my total caloric deficit for each day. ...*sometimes, the journey to success will become inconvenient...*

#2 ADDED IN MORE CARBS, I WAS SLACKING

Previously, I mostly ate carbs in the form of fruit on a regular basis, (unless it was a cheat meal). I realized I needed more satiety to fuel me for my longer days and to help me not cheat in the evenings. I decided to add in a 1/3 rd of a cup of oatmeal for breakfast and 1/2 cup of sweet potato, quinoa, or brown rice at lunch and kept fruit in as a mid-morning snack or afternoon snack (before 4pm) with a protein. Those added carbs kept me sane and encouraged me to stay more focused because I did not feel like I was missing out on a nutrient.

#3 FOOD AS FUEL, NOT AS MY LOVER

Use food as fuel, not for love and affection. During the time I was focused on losing these 10lbs, I was working under three other deadlines. I was attempting to finish writing this book before the end of 2017, finding a new home for my fitness studio, and preparing to head to Tanzania and South Africa for vacation. Scouting locations, reviewing agreements, negotiating contracts, getting vaccines, and assessing moving costs in addition to managing 36 clients, running a studio, making sure I do not start a fire by burning my eggs that are boiling on the stove (I've almost burned the house down twice by doing this SMH), and writing a book is a lot to manage. I do not think anyone would have judge me if I decided to have 3 mimosas, French fries, and 3 brownies during this process because the struggle was *real*. But the truth is, I was not looking for comfort, I was looking for solutions.

Comfort food and alcohol would've physically and mentally slowed down the energy I needed to think under pressure, do research, and get up each day to find a solution to all of these projects. I needed to think clearly, so I ate foods that kept me focused and light on my feet which were fruits, veggies, healthy fats, portion controlled starches and lean proteins. Cravings came but I knew they were a sign of the stress, not the food. When the cravings hit, that is when I assessed my stress and knew I needed some additional nurturing. It was at those times that I proceeded to phone a friend, book an additional hot yoga session, drink another bottle of water, chew gum, take deep breaths, make an effort to go to sleep a little earlier that day, or remind myself why I really need the healthier food as opposed to the Champagne at this time. Nope, not getting off track this time.

#4 NO EXCUSES, YOU'VE RUN OUT OF THEM

I gave myself no excuses. I would say 90% of the time we know what we should be doing to lose weight, we just do not follow through and do it on a consistent basis. This time around, I focused on staying consistent with my meals and meal prepping. If it was not originally on T2's menu, I was not eating or drinking it. Period. I ran out of excuses, options, and situations and chose to stick to my meal prepped foods. I gave myself no other options but to cook what I ate. I did not switch up my meals on the weekend. I either ate what I already meal prepped or purchased to snack on, or chose a healthy option when I went out. I did not allow myself to have the fries just because I was eating out with 4 other people; get real, these people do not know my struggles. I did not buy my obligatory personal birthday cake because I was heading home at 12am; nope, I reminded myself that it was not an option this time. I was not given the authority to order a drink because it was someone else's birthday; I got goals. I did not order a pizza because I had nothing prepared at home. Nah, you better look in that refrigerator one more time and find you a meal. Shoot, especially since you used your hard-earned money buying these foods for your meal prep. I remember one-time making a bootleg 5-minute meal out of hard boiled eggs, hummus, avocado, sugar snap peas, raw broccoli, and blueberries. You were not gonna find me wasting food, wasting money, and gaining weight, oh no honey.

#5 BACK TO BASICS

Back to Basics for me meant drink that water and rest up. I set an alarm on my phone each night at 10:30pm to remind myself to put down my phone and carry my hind parts to bed. I had no business being up later than that and knew it would make me groggy and less focused on being productive in the morning because I would be focused on snacking all day long (true story). In terms of water, I would try to get as close as possible to drinking a half gallon of water. The more water I took in, the more I knew my body would get rid of excess water. I knew my body was responding positively to the additional water because I felt lighter and my stomach "appeared flatter" in a matter of 1 week. So stepping up my water game a bit helped out my weight loss efforts as well.

I ended up losing 3 pounds in the first month and 7 pounds in the second month. You might ask if I followed these 5 steps consistently for those 8 weeks, and the answer is that I followed these rules about 93% of the time. There was that one night in week 3 where I had 2 slices of chocolate cake and 2 glasses of champagne (the rest of the bottle spilled on the floor, so I knew it was sign from the Lord to just stop). I also OD'd on almond butter twice in week 7 (which is way more fat than one should eat in a day). Those mishaps did not affect my overall weight loss because every other time I stuck to my guns. I got back "in the zone" immediately thereafter and was a fat burning machine. The intense bouts of exercises throughout the day (as opposed to concentrated workouts in one session) helped ensure that I was efficiently burning calories throughout the day. I also feel this helped me sleep better. Regardless of the strategies I implemented to drop the 10 pounds, the weight loss would have never happened if I had not figured out a way to get out of my own way. I was getting beat down by life and was in no shape to take on the hardest goal I've ever had to deal with: weight loss. In order to maneuver my way through the fire, over the bridge, and down the hill, I had to put in work by fixing my spirit. Once I fixed my spirit, I was able to embrace the process, patience, and discipline needed to drop the last 10 pounds. I was now someone who lost 100 pounds. Man, this is a phenomenal feeling.

CHAPTER 13

WHAT YOU SHOULD DO TO
LOSE THE LAST 10LBS

LOSING WEIGHT AND maintaining that weight loss is one of the hardest things a person can achieve in life. I'm quite sure you probably feel the same way as I do and are nodding your head as you read this; however, I am a living testimony that it can be done. I do not want to desensitize the issue, overcomplicate weight loss strategies, or sugar coat what is necessary to lose weight in this part of the book. My goal, after all, is truly to help you look at weight loss in a different way so that you can maneuver through those times in the evening or weekends when you just want to give up. I want to give you 10 tips I've used (and am still using) to help lose those last 10 lbs, plus the 90 lbs, I've lost over the years, and how I'm going to continue to maintain this weight loss. The 5 tips I gave you in the previous chapter were essential for cleaning up my specific routine and habits so I could get over that plateau. The next 10 tips I want to leave you with are crucial if you've noticed you keep starting your weight loss journey over and over and do not know how to start again, how to stick with it, or how to maintain it. You might also be looking for a guide to assist you with dropping your own last 10 lbs and do not know where to begin. This section is for you. My goal is to keep this portion of the book as simple (but thorough) as possible. So to help me help you wherever you are in your weight loss journey, I'm going to talk to you just like I talk to my clients, which means no BS.

USE SOCIAL MEDIA FOR INSPIRATION, NOT DUPLICATION

Assess the landscape and use it for inspiration, not duplication. Whether you are attempting to lose those last 10 lbs or needing to commit to a healthier lifestyle, you must understand what is happening on a macro and micro level around you and see what role that is playing on your psyche. We are currently living in a fast-paced, technologically driven, highlight reel society. We pick up our phone a hundred times a day and every time we do, it gives us instant access to so much information, including pictures and videos on weight loss transformations, new weight loss trends, new food diets, new 30-day weight loss challenges, new workout equipment, and uber-fit women in all age groups with a 24 inch waist and 42 inch hips. As a woman, I know that we are all guilty of judging other women, obsessing over things we do not like about our body, and wanting to emulate the body and lifestyle of other women in some sort of fashion.

I gotta tell you right now, to lose this weight, you cannot compare yourself to someone else because 9 times out of 10, you are going to negatively critique yourself, not the other person, and this is going to affect your level of motivation. Stalking someone else's life on social media, your coworker who somehow naturally lost 42 lbs in 4 months, or following any and every weight loss trend that hits the market gets into your brain and in your spirit and can be mentally draining. This obsession takes away from the focus and effort you could be using for real and permanent change, but instead it keeps you stuck in neutral. Let's look at the facts: every woman's body loses weight at different rates, in different areas, and has a different chemical makeup from your sister, BFF, girlfriend, or your "friend" on Facebook that looks like she drops 7lbs every friggin' week. We are all different, get over it! Remember, it took me 2 years to lose weight (not 6 months). It's a high probability you will never look like the women next to you, but I guaranteed if you took the focus off the Instagram girl with the 2 pack abs and put it into your own routine, plenty of people would think you have a banging body as well. Use social media, television, and movies to inspire you to stay consistent, not to emulate other women. I guarantee you could probably do better than the next woman if 1) you truly put your mind to it and 2) remember they went through (and are currently going through) the same issues as you are behind the scenes, it just did not make their highlight reel (i.e. Facebook/Instagram post).

DO YOU BELIEVE YOU CAN DO IT?

Assess how your past has shaped your behaviors, beliefs, feelings, and actions toward losing weight. Think hard on this one, "What are your thoughts about the fact that you've failed 726 times in the past at losing weight?" Do you believe that despite all of those failures you can still lose weight? Do you think you are unable to lose weight because you are over 50 years, over 275 lbs, have a thyroid issue, you have been big boned since you were 3 years old, you have a busy schedule, you are the mother of a special needs child, and you have never lost more than 20 lbs at once in your lifetime? In order to lose weight, YOU must be your strongest ally. You must love yourself enough to want more than what you presently have or how far you have gone in the past. You have gotta stop the self-sabotage once you lose 20 lbs for the 4th time in your life; instead, you must have an intense desire to see what it feels like to lose 26 lbs this time around. If you have doubt and are betting against yourself once you start your weight loss routine, you will eventually fail. In fact, you will epically fail. Every single day on your weight loss journey, you are gonna have to put two feet on the floor and make the decision all day long to stay committed; that is the only way you will lose weight. You are going to have to stick it out even though you are not "feeling it" and/or if your best friend or your husband is doing something totally different. Despite the odds, you must do and you must believe in YOU. If you ain't feeling that type of effort right now, then I do not suggest you start because you are going to get your little feelings hurt. You have to be selfish (which in this instance is a great thing) and DO YOU in order to lose weight. Still take care of your other responsibilities, but if you are not willing to move yourself up the priority chain, please have several seats.

BE REALISTIC ABOUT YOUR METHODS FOR WEIGHT LOSS

Reassess your goals in a realistic fashion. Please do not be out here trying to lose weight just for a season. Ain't nobody got time to just look cute for one month! We gotta stop with the yo-yo dieting and stick to the basics as much as possible. So that means no more diet teas, waist trainers, 10-day smoothie diets, weekly detoxes, weight loss pills and prescription medications, Cool Sculpting, waist sweat bands, etc. Check with your friends who have tried these quick fixes. Remember what they said and what happened when you followed the guidelines step by step with these weight loss trends? What happened? More than likely, you either lost a little weight, did not lose weight at all, started to experience some side effects, or did not stick with it because you were not seeing any results or it was a drastic change from your current lifestyle. These short-term weight loss fixes are not doing anything to get to the root of the issue of why you are not losing weight and is not something you can maintain over your lifetime. You gonna still wear a waist trainer for 10 hours a day at 53 years old? When you attempt to lose the weight this time around, please be upfront with yourself about what you realistically can achieve in 3 months, 6 months, and 9 months. Take into account your work and family responsibilities and see what you can honestly give to yourself to make this weight loss a reality. Progress takes patience. We have our whole lives ahead of us, so do not put unnecessary time frames on when you should lose 30lbs. As long as you are putting in quality effort, just stay focused on maintaining the environment, habits, and actions necessary for change to take place on a consistent basis. Once you do that, the weight will come off on its own.

RESTRUCTURE YOUR FOCUS

Commit to restructuring your thoughts, behaviors, and habits that are in line to reach your goals. Do not think, complain, vent, and moan that you have to go through "all of this" just to lose weight. So freaking what! Don't you jump through hoops to get a good deal on some Beyoncé concert tickets? Was it you that just planned an epic girls trip for you and your girls to Essence Festival last year? What about the cute jumpsuit you religiously waited 4 weeks to purchase because you know at 2:55pm on Thursday, October 14th they are going to put their clothes on sale for 40% off? Didn't you find a way to take care of your husband, make it to both of your kids' basketball games all season long after work, and still manage to finish graduate school with get a 3.5 GPA? Ok? Do not act like you are unaccustomed to putting in work for a sweet reward or surprise. You will go out of your way to research, scout, travel, and purchase far and wide to get some awesome things done for your family and friends, but you mean to tell me you are not going to do that for your body (which by the way, we only get one of in this lifetime)? Come on, now! This body will fail you when you forget to pay attention to it. So I need you to transfer the same energy you put into other people, events, and things into yourself to receive change. Stop sulking and just put in the work.

I would also like to mention that if you feel you are giving your all and things are not working as you think they should, then I suggest you make every effort to find out what is the culprit and that includes on a medical level as well. As women we tend to have hormonal issues that could also play a role in our weight loss efforts. Our bodies change as we get older, so even though you have been eating healthy on a regular basis, you may now find out you need additional fiber in your diet that you were not previously getting in the past. You may need to increase the dosage of your iron supplement you have been taking for the past 4 years. You may have to reduce the amount of fruit you are eating because your body is not absorbing sugar properly and it is staying longer in your blood stream. With body changes such as these occurring regularly as we get older, I highly suggest taking a trip to your MD and OBGYN. Before starting a fitness/weight loss program, it is important that you ask your doctor to give you a blood test and a hormone panel test that includes checking your estrogen, progesterone, as well as your thyroid level. Most imbalances can be corrected by adding and removing certain foods out of your diet as well as taking in certain herbs, while others might require you to take a pill. You will not know what move to take unless you start looking at the glass half full as opposed to half empty, so fix your attitude and take yourself to the doctor (*sometimes there is more to it than diet and exercise*). You can make time for your body.

TAKE YOUR FEELINGS OUT OF THE EQUATION

We have got to become in-tune with our body and that requires us to put effort into finding out what we truly need to seek change. In this regard, it's less about how you feel and more about how you move. If getting in your workouts and eating healthy from week to week only happened if you "feel like doing it," you will never experience real results. Just like if you always ate junk food or drank alcohol every single time you felt like it, you would probably be bigger than you are at this moment. Take your friggin' feelings out of it! No, you don't get 4 cookies every single time you had a "long day" or you made it to the weekend. Feelings are not always truths and will lead you onto a dead end with no weight loss in sight. This time on your weight loss journey you need to shift your focus from feelings to action. When that thought comes in to your mind, 'I should get up and go to the gym,' or 'You know what, it is nice outside I should go for a walk'...DO IT! You also need to move when you get home and you are feeling blah, got an attitude because of your boss at work, or just plain tired from the day and you are itching to reward yourself with certain foods or drinks. Take a walk, take an extra jog around the neighborhood, get in some push-ups, or take your frustrations out on a treadmill, instead of raising your blood sugar levels again (with foods and drinks our bodies have no use for) and increasing your body's fat storage abilities. Our bodies were not made to sit all day long at work, then drive home (sitting), sit on the couch (sitting), go to sleep (lying down), then do the same thing day after day. NAH. Deal with your feelings by being active, not sedentary. Don't give up.

EVEN ON YOUR WORST DAY, DON'T GIVE UP!

Giving up on yourself means there is a 100% chance you will not reach your goals. Period. You have essentially taken yourself out of the running for transformation if you quit. So this time around, whatever you do, DON'T GIVE UP. If you cannot put in 60 minutes at the gym because you are running the kids back and forth to football practice, do 22 minutes around the track while they are practicing and call it a day. If your lunch choice sucked, pick up the healthy eating at dinner, not next Monday. Let me let you in on a little secret. Oftentimes, the people end up losing weight are the ones who stick with it longer than the people who give up...that is it! It is not the person who has more free time than you, or a gym in their home, or a personal trainer, or a chef, or the woman who happens to be smaller than you. None of that really matters. What matters is whether you recognize the urgency in not giving up on yourself from week to week. So instead of quitting at 3 months and 4 days, push it to 4 whole months and see what it feels like to stay consistent for a longer period of time. Just barely staying on the course will help you develop more consistency, better self confidence, and more healthy habits. This will get you quicker to the finish line than the chick who called for security to pick her up at mile 2...DON'T GIVE UP!!!

BE FAIR, BUT FIRM TO YOURSELF

Develop a routine that is realistic, works with your schedule, yet is challenging enough to invoke change and something that you can maintain on a weekly basis. To date, I've trained over 1600 men and women in Hampton Roads and online. My clients have ranged from 13 years old to 93 years old. I've trained people that have gone through back surgery, 2 heart surgeries, all types of cancers, knee replacements, hip replacements, pacemaker in place, recently divorced, going through a divorce, was mentally hospitalized that same year, etc. All of these clients were experiencing a combination of residual effects because of these conditions, which obviously had an impact in addition to their busy schedules. My clients' occupations consist of being home health aides, administrative assistants, doctors, teachers, social workers, nurses, attorneys, students, accountants, and waitresses, all while taking care of their 2 to 3 kids and finishing up their master's degree at night. So, you being busy ain't nothing new, chile. No one is at home twiddling their thumbs; everyone is getting home late, dropping off and picking up people, running back and forth to this appointment, checking in on friends, all while still trying to stay sane. That being said, stop with the excuses (there will always be at least 5 excuses you could give yourself a day), and let's devise a firm strategy to drop this weight once and for all.

GET ORGANIZED

Take out a sheet of paper and write down all the days of the week at the top of the page and leave room on the rest of the page to write in your work schedule, kids appointments, meetings, travel, and your personal appointments. Next, write in what days and times you have left to workout. Remember, your exercise time could be 10 minutes Tuesday afternoon, 30 minutes Monday night, 60 minutes Sunday afternoon; just write in what times you can commit to training. We know that life takes us on twists and turns, so you MUST be flexible enough to change the days and times of your workouts if other "important" responsibilities come up from week to week. (Replacement workouts to do at home are clutch for keeping the mind in line with your goals if you cannot make it to class or the gym.) Do not get caught up in the idea that you can only workout at a certain time of day. The best time to work out is when you actually make it to working out, so roll with that motto from now on. Once you put it in the planner, do not allow frivolous alternatives to dissuade you from working out...*goals over excuses!* If you are not already utilizing strength or resistance training as a part of your fitness routine, add it in, chile! As I mentioned earlier, strength training is an important way to help you reduce body fat and increase your metabolism (the rate at which your body burns fuel). Just doing cardiovascular exercise alone will not help the body to change shape, improve your strength (which is needed as we get older), develop muscle tone, and help you burn additional calories when you are chilling watching TV; you need strength training in your fitness routine for those type of results. Do not fear the weight, honey! Also, keep those workouts fun and challenging! Keep the fun workouts around for those days when you do not feel like exercising but you know once you get there you are gonna have a great time.

Another point to remember about workouts is that if your workouts do not challenge you, they will not change you. It does you no good to do the same weak circuit you have been doing at the gym for the past 6 months or the same Zumba routine each week that you could teach the class yourself. Step it up! Feel the extra soreness on your joints and the increased sweat from a more challenging workout; your body can take it and build you up to be an even stronger fat-burning machine. At the same time, do not start working out 7 days a week doing Olympic lifting, cross fit, and spinning and then you stop exercising altogether because you knew goodness well you could not keep up with that level of activity. If your body is used to working out, focus on staying consistent with working out while increasing the intensity of your workouts via an increased resistance load, more High Intensity Interval Training (HIIT) exercises, and/or sprints while performing cardiovascular activity. Start where you are and build from there, but be realistic about where you are along your fitness journey.

In addition to getting organized with your workout regimen, you must put effort into developing a better relationship with food. As humans, eating is the number one activity we have to do several times of day. We can easily eat 4-6 times a day, 7 days a week. We need to develop a relationship with food that is healthy, nurturing, and supportive of our busy lifestyles. We should be eating to provide fuel for our busy lifestyles and crazy schedules (which also means we need to eat even if you are busy), not to solve any personal, career, and family issues that come up along "The Journey." I encourage everyone to try your darnedest to be present when you eat. You are choosing to eat healthy meals and snacks because you are responsible for taking care of your body, not because you are on punishment. We should enjoy "cheat meals" at times, but not at the expense of abusing (overeating) our body. Choosing healthier options when dealing with the demands of life on a daily basis, becomes difficult when we wait until the last minute to decide what we are going to eat. Prepping your food is the best way to provide fuel, order, productivity, and structure to your life. As I mentioned earlier, meal prepping will also save you time, money, and calories each and every week. So make the effort for one to two hours on Sundays to plan out your meals. Get it together!

GET ONGOING HELP TO STAY CONSISTENT

One of the reasons I became a personal trainer is so I could help people devise a strategy to reach their weight loss goals wherever they are in life. We are quick to get the plumber to fix our toilet, the mechanic to fix our car, and sometimes you might need a personal trainer to help you fix your fitness lifestyle (or lack thereof). Questions can be answered, motivation can be provided, accountability can be checked and workouts can be devised to challenge your body for more change than you would have got on your own or doing it with your fitness friend. That being said, assess whether you need a personal trainer, nutritionist, or mental therapist to assist you along your weight loss journey. You cannot be afraid to ask for help; we do not know everything and at this moment, we need all hands on deck to help you be awesome.

NO "DIETS" ALLOWED, JUST EAT REAL FOOD

The final tip I want to say about developing a realistic routine has to do with how we eat. Every 1-2 years, a new diet comes around that everyone and their momma is looking to try out since it is touted by health critics as the next best thing. (By the time you read this book, a new food trend would have probably made its way into the world.) When I started on my weight loss journey, the low-fat diet was considered the best way to lose weight. Nowadays, you have about 6-8 diets rolling around to confuse the bejesus out of all us as the best way to lose weight. Some of the trendy diets out right now include The Paleo Diet, The Vegan Diet, The Ketogenic Diet, The Atkins Diet, The Mediterranean

Diet, Carb Cycling, Intermittent Fasting, Juicing/ Blending, Flexible Dieting, The DASH diet, If It Fits Your Macros Diet (IIFYM), etc. I'm not going to go in to any detail about these diets because that is enough information for an entirely different book. I think there is an incentive to incorporating any of these diets/nutritional strategies/eating patterns into your routine. I also believe they could assist you to lose weight, but I'm just not sure if it is the best way to approach weight loss from a long-term perspective. I do not even know you, but I know it is impossible for you to juice all of your meals for the rest of your life. For some people, it may be difficult to count the calories of your meals every single day to keep up with Carb Cycling on a long-term basis. Intermittent Fasting can be a good way to drop some unnecessary pounds and fat, but do you really think you can go 16 hours every day without eating food for 365 days a year? Do not over-complicate the task of choosing healthy food options on a regular basis and get into a yo-yo dieting routine; it can wreak havoc on the body in more ways than one.

My advice: Do not try to come up with a label for how you eat. For all intents and purposes, people would put me into the category of pescatarian, but I do not necessarily look at myself in that way, and you should not worry about putting yourself into a certain category either. My focus is on consistently choosing healthy proteins to maintain my muscle mass and definition, high fiber foods to keep my digestive system working effectively (and helps to keep my waist snatched), keeping my sugar and alcohol intake low to keep my blood sugar normalized, and getting in as many vegetables as I can to keep antioxidants high, hormones balanced, and providing me all the vitamins and minerals my body needs on a daily basis. When I put the focus on planning out (and meal prepping) healthy foods instead of choosing a specific diet, it helped me feel less restricted and more in-tune to the needs of my body. Fueling your body properly should be the focus, not whether you have been "going Paleo for 8 months." Focus on the food, (not the labels of food diets) and the rest will take care of the body on its own.

Furthermore, our diet consists of whatever goes into your stomach, so you need to focus on cleaning up your diet on a consistent basis rather than focusing on adapting to the newest diet on the market. Completing your workouts and choosing healthy food options can already be a hard pill to swallow, so do not pile it on with specialty diets. Do your research on the pros and cons for eating animal proteins, dairy, raw and cooked vegetables, alcohol, sugar (including natural sugar) and listen and feel how your body responds to these foods. The food amount and type of nutrients can play a significant role in whether or not you are dropping weight. Raw vegetables and dairy tend to disrupt the digestive process for some people, which can affect the metabolism, so you may need to keep those at bay. As I mentioned earlier, my body does not approve of the use of alcohol, sugar and processed carbs (sometimes even healthy ones), so I keep those limited. If you are used to eating healthy and feel advanced in the health and fitness game, then you may want to try Carb Cycling or Intermittent Fasting, as these eating patterns have been known to help some people burn additional fat. If you are like, "Look, I'm just trying to stay on the wagon this time around," then do not over-complicate it and keep the food simple.

Since I ended my journey losing 100 pounds, I will not sit here and say, "You know looking back, losing the weight was actually an easy thing." Get real. Like I've said several times during this book, losing weight and maintaining that weight loss for the past 15 years is the hardest thing I've had to do in life. Anyone that tells you losing weight is easy must be an alien and they do not know our struggles. But even though it is the most difficult thing I've had to do, I'ma tell you this: it can be done for you as well. There is no difference between you or I in our journey towards living a better life. Losing 100 lbs was more about gaining control of my life as opposed to watching it pass me by. To gain control of my life, I had to hit rock bottom and then one level below that in order for me to get rid of the excuses, bad habits, pity, grief, and victim mentality that kept me there. Once I committed to being an active participant in my life, the pitfalls, booby traps, and roadblocks were no match for the conviction flowing through my veins. I started to be an advocate for myself as opposed to a dependent. My self-love improved, I went to therapy and I started to seek ways to put positive physical and mental effort into my spirit. By changing my mental landscape, it created the perfect platform for me to conceptualize the ultimate weight loss strategy for myself. My mental game was so clear that I was able to get in the zone, devise the best strategy to make healthy food choices on a daily basis given my busy schedule, all while taking the pressure off of me that was holding me back for all these years. Once the weight started to come off, I maintained my weight loss by remembering the purpose of food as well as embodying the patience, discipline, and workout habits necessary to make them fully become a part of my lifestyle.

If you made it to the end of this book with me, please know that every day you wake up means you have been given another day to gain control of your life. WAKE UP! YOU MATTER! Likewise, your thoughts, feelings, actions, and eating habits should reflect how much you love and matter to yourself on a regular basis. Every single day, every single hour, every single meal you are able to partake in means you have been given the task to make a choice. Do you feel that you have the power at 42 years old to make a change each day? You must believe. If you do not believe, I encourage you to find the "WHY" for why YOU are living. Even with the running back and forth with kids, taking care of a sick parent, being in school, going to work, you still MUST take care of yourself. Making it a priority to take care of yourself should not be looked at as being selfish. You have noticed in the past that when you decide to make healthy food choices, get in those workouts, get in proper sleep, check in with your doctor and treat yourself as the awesome person you already are, the order and less stress that comes your way starts to carry over to other areas of your life. When more order (discipline) is established in your routine, you function better at work, at home, and with your family and friends. Am I right?

So stop allowing yourself unhealthy options (when that is not what you REALLY want) and recognize the power of utilizing energy and effort specifically to enhance our well-being: you matter! People who are in relationships and marriages have to recommit each day to stay with their spouse, because the truth is you can leave; it may be hard to leave or you might feel like leaving is not an option, but you have a choice. The same should be said for the relationship you have with yourself. Shift your actions to recommitting every day to this lifestyle with no other options available. Stop trying to leave all the got dag on time! Even if you had one small slice of pizza at Keisha's son's birthday party, do not take it to the next level with more food, happy hour shenanigans, and late-night binge eating. Instead of trying to leave yourself, believe that you will pick back up the healthy eating at your next meals (one slice of pizza will not kill your progress). This type of strength will not be developed until you become patient with the fact that you have to recommit each day. Willpower is not infinite. It runs out very quickly, so you must be willing to help remove barriers that can stop you from getting into the zone (i.e. bring healthy snacks with you, eat before you leave the house, drink enough water, read your Bible if you are a believer, talk to your accountability partner, etc.) everyday. You have to continue to pour into yourself every day to get the outcome in which you have been yearning for years. Because holding on to the pizza, the alcohol, the sugar, the negative self-talk, and the toxic relationships will not truly satisfy you the way weight loss will. You want to lose those last 10 lbs, right? So fix your face, fix that funky little attitude, breathe, and make the choice each day to give your body what it needs and not what it wants. I dare you to make this a habit and see what happens! Stop waiting to "feel good" about exercising, choosing healthier options, or starting a new routine. At this very moment, you have the power within you to give your mind and body the order, patience, discipline, and love it needs to lose the weight, so do it now. *RIGHT NOW*!

SUGGESTED READING LIST

I realize that a number of factors can have a favorable or unfavorable impact along your weight loss journey; so I've compiled a reading list that addresses some of the issues people usually face (including myself) along "The Journey" that I could not discuss in detail in the book. The focus of content in this reading list is to not only help you reach those fitness goals once and for all, but more importantly maintain those results for the long-term. So please check out any of the books below if you feel that they are applicable to where you are along your journey. Happy reading!

Amidor, Toby. The Healthy Meal Prep Cookbook. Easy and Wholesome Meals to Cook, Prep, Grab and Go. Rockridge Press. 2017

Campbell, Adam. The Women's Health Big Book of Exercises: Four Weeks to a Leaner, Sexier, Healthier You. Rodale Books. 2016.

Duhigg, Charles. The Power of Habit. Why We Do What We do In Life and In Business. New York: Random House Trade Paperbacks. 2012.

Frankel, Bethenny. Naturally Thin. New York: Fireside Trade Paperbacks Edition. 2009.

Gaesser, Glenn, PH.D. Big Fat Lies: The Truth About Your Weight and Health. Canada: Ballentine Books. 1996.

Tumminello, Nick. Strength Training For Fat Loss. Human Kinetics. 2014.

Wansink, Brian. Mindless Eating: Why We Eat More Than We Think. Bantam Publishing. 2006.

Wolever, Ruth, PHD. The Mindful Diet: How to Transform Your Relationship with Food For Lasting Weight Loss and Vibrant Health. Scribner Publishing. 2016.

BIOGRAPHY

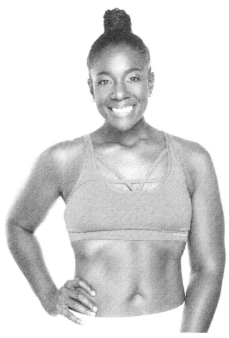

Tasha Turnbull is a certified personal trainer, group fitness instructor, fitness nutrition specialist, motivational speaker and an award winning entrepreneur. She owns T2 Fitness Studios, a fitness training facility in Virginia Beach, Va. Tasha has spoken on several radio stations in the Hampton Roads area. She has also been featured on several television shows in Hampton Roads as well as a nationally syndicated television show. She has been a personal trainer for 9 years and a fitness studio owner for 7 years. She currently lives in Virginia Beach, Va.

Made in the USA
Coppell, TX
06 February 2021

49796375R00125